American Nursing And The Failed Dream

A Critical Assessment Of Nursing Education In America

JUNE M. HARRINGTON

ISBN: 1-4392-3568-6
ISBN-13: 9781439235683
LCCN: 2009903176

Visit www.booksurge.com to order additional copies.

A special thanks
to my nephew F. Dean Harrington
for his encouragement and support for this endeavor

Dedication
The Class of 1958
St. Joseph's Hospital School of Nursing
Providence, Rhode Island

CONTENTS

Introduction ix

1 A House in Chaos 1

2 In the Beginning 11

3 Enter Lady Reformers 23

4 Groundwork for a Big Problem 35

5 In Context 51

6 Standards First, Country Second 71

7 Some Defining Moments 91

8 More Reports, More Recalcitrance 109

9 Mildred's Misconception 123

10 The '60s, the '70s, and the Professional Issue 139

11 Counsel from the Past 153

12 Who Speaks for Thee? 179

13 The Shortage Thing 199

14 Always a Bridesmaid 217

INTRODUCTION

This narrative is my perspective regarding nursing education in America. My intent is to explain to the reader why I believe the education of American nurses is not on course. I am speaking as a nurse about nursing. Consequently, the reader should know something of my nursing background.

In September 1955, I entered as a student nurse into the three-year hospital diploma program at St. Joseph's Hospital in Providence, Rhode Island. My experience was apprenticeship training at its best. Student nurses of this era, like so many generations before them, were the workhorses of the nursing service. We provided most of the direct nursing care to patients. The work was laborious, and the responsibility charged to girls who were too young to vote was, by today's ethical standards, highly questionable. However, this apprenticeship training provided a working-class girl with a vocation and assisted in keeping hospital costs for patients at a minimum. Student nurses received room, board, and experience.

The timeframe was mid-twentieth-century America, and the three-year hospital diploma nursing educational programs produced the largest number of graduate nurses in the U.S.

The first segment of the program of about six months was referred to as the preclinical period. We were special students at Providence College, where we studied basic anatomy, physiology, chemistry, and social sciences. We referred to these courses as "pressure cooker" courses. They were characterized by brief and intensive instruction. The remaining two and one-half years was spent in different clinical areas of the hospital and other health agencies. Classroom instruction was now primarily disease oriented. There was a three-month psychiatric affiliation at the state hospital, an eight-week affiliation at a communicable disease hospital, and an eight-week affiliation at a visiting nurse agency. I found the psychiatric affiliation the most rewarding of my student clinical experiences. There was an eight-week experience in the operating room, and this presented a great opportunity to learn human anatomy. In the operating room, you could see and sometimes feel the organs of the human body. You see, student nurses did not dissect a human cadaver, as did medical students. Student nurses learned their anatomy by dissecting the domestic cat.

One day I was assigned to scrub for a major abdominal case. The patient had an intestinal cancer. At a certain point the surgeon determined the cancer had spread to the liver. The surgeon and other members of the surgical team discussed the probable negative outcome for the anesthetized patient. I was diligently holding an abdominal retractor, trying my best to get a look into the patient's abdominal cavity. The surgeon said, "Give me your hand. I want you to feel this." He navigated my hand over the patient's liver, and I actually felt the disease process that was consuming this vital organ. "That, young lady, is cancer," he said. That was also an example of the on-the-spot, unstructured, learn-as-you-go process characteristic of the three-year hospital diploma program.

In September 1958, I graduated and was a recipient of the Mother Evangelist Scholarship Award in recognition of scholastic achievement, professional leadership, and nursing performance. In November I passed the state board examination for licensure as a registered nurse (RN).

I migrated to Boston and assumed a position as staff nurse at Massachusetts General Hospital. Boston was the home of major teaching hospitals, major medical schools, and several four-year collegiate nursing programs. In terms of nursing education, the time spent in Boston increased my awareness of the declining prestige of hospital diploma programs. Many in nursing, particularly nurse educators, did not consider graduates of these programs to be professional nurses. They believed the hospital program was too technically focused, and only a nurse with a formal academic background could render professional nursing care.

In the fall 1959, I became a full-time student at Boston College. The School of Nursing had a two-year completion program for RNs from diploma schools of nursing. Their policy was to award college credit for clinical experience obtained in the basic program. While the RN student took a few clinical courses, the majority of the credit hours

were earned in the arts and sciences. The time spent
at Boston College was rewarding in all aspects. It was
somewhat expensive. I paid the first semester's tuition with
scholarship money I received at graduation from
St. Joseph's and obtained National Student Defense Loans.
I managed everyday expenses by "specialing" on weekends
and holidays. You placed your name with a registry and
specified which of the Boston hospitals you would like
for a patient assignment. The utilization of special nurses,
sometimes called private duty nurses, was one way the
Boston hospitals dealt with their chronic nursing shortage.
I was one of many in the Boston area who were graduates
of diploma programs, going to school on a full-time basis,
working part time, just making it financially. Most of us
were in our twenties, and we experienced a strong sense
of camaraderie. We did not believe we graduated from
inferior nursing programs. However, we were realistic.
The baccalaureate degree was a basic requirement for
career growth.

The 1960s was a time of turmoil and change. It brought
the Kennedy assassinations, the Vietnam War, the Women's
Movement, student uprisings, and extraordinary medical
advances. Concomitantly, the American nursing leadership
was expending their energy on one particular issue. They
were trying to convince anyone who would listen that the
nurses from collegiate nursing programs were the one and
only true professional nurses. While most of the turmoil
of the '60s found some level of resolution, the turmoil
within American nursing about the professional issue was
gaining momentum.

I decided to pursue advanced education in the clinical area that provided me with the greatest satisfaction.

In 1964, I began the master's degree program in adult psychiatric nursing at New York University. The financial burdens of my Boston era were in the past. The federal government would pay tuition and provide a substantial monthly stipend to RNs who studied to be clinical nurse specialists in psychiatric nursing. My tuition was paid in full to one of the largest private universities in America.

I was living in New York City. I had access to such nursing notables as Martha Rogers, Dorothy Mereness, Claire Fagin, and Jesse Mae Pepper. The academic program was rigorous. The clinical affiliations included some of the largest psychiatric facilities in New York. New York had it all. New York also increased my awareness of the professional issue and its penetrating impact on academic nurses, the major constituents of the nursing establishment.

In 1965, the American Nurses Association (ANA) published a very important paper on nursing education. In nursing circles it became known as the "Position Paper" and will be discussed in Chapter 10 of this narrative. The paper identified the baccalaureate degree in nursing as the professional degree. This single publication created havoc within American nursing. It relegated the majority of RNs to non-professional status. In some cases it put nurses in opposition to one another. It separated nurses according to their basic nursing education. It challenged the very heart and soul of American nursing. I was still at NYU, bearing witness to the hubris of nurse academics who were the major advocates of this paper. They were certain they had finally put American nursing on the path to *professionhood*. They were wrong.

I received my master's degree in June 1966. The period at NYU would complete my formal academic preparation in nursing. Following NYU, I engaged in a number of pursuits. I was a psychiatric clinical nurse specialist, an assistant director of nurses in a psychiatric hospital, an associate professor of psychiatric nursing in a two-year associate degree program, and an assistant director of a three-year hospital diploma program. In 1976, I joined the Department of Veterans Affairs and remained with the organization until retirement in December 1997. My initial position was as an instructor in nursing education. In this position I dealt directly with the extensive orientation and inservice needs of new graduate nurses from all types of nursing educational programs—BSN, ADN, diploma and practical nursing programs. I also held the position of associate chief nurse for education, assistant chief nurse, and chief nurse. By assuming the latter two positions, I was changing from an educational focus to the administration of a nursing service.

My years in nursing administration were the most rewarding and enlightening in terms of problems within nursing. Part of my enlightenment came via educationally unprepared graduate nurses, chronic nursing shortages, and a variety of staffing issues as perceived by the nurse, hospital administrators, nursing supervisors, and representatives of labor unions. As I neared retirement I realized many critical issues in American nursing remained unresolved. Most of these critical issues had been around as long as I had been in nursing. Like me, they were simply getting old. What is the problem with American nursing? I thought it an appropriate post-retirement endeavor to study this question. I did a great deal of research and found answers. My conclusion is the problems in American nursing originated with the professional issue—the failed dream. The following chapters will provide the details.

June M. Harrington

1

A HOUSE IN CHAOS

The house of American nursing is not in order. Poorly defined nursing education, a chronic nursing shortage, and the lack of effective nursing leadership are three major issues that threaten the very existence of the Nightingale concept of nursing in the United States. American nursing is bordering on implosion. If this occurs, like the phoenix, a new category of healthcare worker will rise from the ashes. Only a change in the mindset of nursing leaders and major changes in nursing education will alter this outcome.

There are nearly three million individuals in the U.S. with the title Registered Nurse (RN). The majority acquired their basic nursing education in two-year associate degree programs offered by junior or community colleges. Most of the remaining received their basic nursing education in four-year baccalaureate programs at colleges or universities. Regardless of where they supposedly learned their elementary nursing skills, at graduation students of neither program were prepared to assume the basic duties of a staff nurse in an in-patient setting.

Interestingly this disturbing fact is not a secret. New graduates and their employers know this. Nursing professors know this. State boards of nursing know this. National nursing organizations know this. Probably the only people who do not know this are future students of nursing and the American taxpayer. The latter still provides substantial financial support to nursing education.

What is the significance of these realities? First, in-patient facilities remain the largest employer of nurses and rely on the two- and four-year colleges to provide these nurses. Second, at considerable expense, in-patient facilities must provide extensive on-the-job training for new graduate nurses. The fact is basic nursing educational programs preparing students for licensure as registered nurses are simply not relevant. They are generic in nature and do not focus on nursing skills needed in the in-patient setting. Is the process of educating nurses on target to meet the needs of American society? The answer is an emphatic "no."

There is the issue of the omnipresent nursing shortage. Catastrophic nursing shortages have been predicted by the nursing leadership since the conclusion of WWII. This is well documented in the nursing literature. The nursing leadership generally employs a two-pronged approach to the problem. First, the U.S. Congress is petitioned for additional money for the education of additional nurses. Second, and with the help of the general media, the public is kept well informed of nurses' general discontent, disenchantment, and disdain with working conditions in the in-patient setting. The general media provides considerable information via newspaper accounts, non-fiction narratives, professional journals, and magazine articles. The generally accepted reasons for the situation have remained consistent throughout the years. Give nurses more money, more respect, every weekend off, no mandatory overtime, and state-regulated staffing guidelines. These proposals have been tried, yet the chronic nursing shortage and unhappiness of American nurses remains unabated. These efforts only address symptoms of what is ailing American nursing. The reality is the underlying problem is complex in nature, intangible, quite serious, and caused by the manner in which nurses are educated and not the manner in which they are treated. Why has the nursing leadership failed to address this basic issue? The answer may surprise you.

Who comprises the nursing leadership in the U.S.? To whom or to what entity can American society turn for answers about nursing education and practice? The fact is American nursing leadership is diffuse in nature. This has had a devastating effect on the largest segment of healthcare workers in the U.S. Also, this is a major contributing factor to the inability of American nursing to resolve many long-standing issues such as the chronic nursing shortage. Absent is a contemporary nursing leader of significant stature who can speak for the majority of American nurses. There is not available one body, council, or organization to represent the composite interests of American nurses. There are close to three million nurses in the U.S., yet American nursing is not a significant force on the national scene, politically or otherwise. Close to three million strong yet nurses in the U.S. lack the necessary cohesiveness to formulate a game plan to ensure survival in the twenty-first century. Is the answer a national nursing oversight council?

Modern American nursing made its debut in the mid-1860s under the auspices of the Civil War. Following the war some members of this new vocation moved from the battlefield into the home as private duty nurses. Others became essential members of the evolving hospital scene. However, a general discontent emerged among late nineteenth and early twentieth century nursing leaders. They became increasingly concerned about the work status and societal perception of the nurse. It was the reactions of the early nursing leaders and their successors to these concerns that essentially subverted nursing education in America. The leaders believed, in order to improve the work situation and societal image of nurses, the vocation of nursing should be raised to the level of a profession. This would require a higher level of education for the nurse, which was eventually identified as the collegiate level. Also, higher education would attract the "right kind of woman" to the ranks of American nursing. This belief system influenced American nursing well into the twentieth century. Attempting to make nursing a profession became an end unto itself. It became the "why" behind the ineffectiveness of American nursing education. It is the reason the United States cannot maintain a stable nursing workforce. It is the essential factor supporting the divisiveness among American nurses. It is the author's opinion that advocates of this belief system, past and present, constitute the de facto nursing establishment.

Prior to the 1970s, the majority of nurses were trained (and that is the correct term) in three-year hospital diploma programs. The hospital ward was the classroom and the student nurse was the apprentice worker who provided nursing care to patients. The head nurse or staff nurses provided oversight of the student's performance. There was some classroom instruction, but clinical experience was the primary method of learning. The student nurse was an essential component of hospital staffing. She was considered a financial asset. Eventually the majority of hospital diploma programs closed.

Four-year college/university programs and two-year community/junior college programs assumed the educational responsibility for preparing nurses for the workplace. Ultimately the two-year junior/community college program became the major provider of new graduate nurses in the U.S. The curriculum and clinical experiences of the two- and four-year programs differed substantially from each other and from the few remaining three-year hospital programs. However, the two- and four-year programs had two commonalities. Both programs resided in institutions of higher learning and both programs significantly curtailed the student's hospital clinical experience in favor of a liberal arts education. As the liberal arts subjects assumed a greater portion of the nursing curriculum, fewer hours were allocated to in-patient clinical areas as sites for students' learning experiences.

By design, nursing educational programs changed substantially and the impact was significant. A new era in nursing education had emerged. Over time the operational and practical aspects of nursing in the in-patient setting received substantially less attention in the nursing curriculum. Consequently and over time these critical elements were not developed in the curriculum, and nursing curriculums failed to meet the demands of an evolving high-technology hospital setting. Thus the majority of graduating nurses were unprepared, emotionally and technically, to assume the position of a beginning nurse in the in-patient setting.

This situation remains to this day. New graduates of both programs require an extraordinary degree of mentoring, skill enhancement and supervision—all at the employers' expense. Nursing educational programs have become irrelevant in terms of meeting the educational needs of the student preparing to work in an in-patient setting. The four-year college/university programs are generic in nature. The focus of the curriculum is eclectic as reflected in descriptive phases as "nursing patients in multiple settings," "nursing of patients throughout the life span," or "nursing along the health/disease continuum." The two-year junior/community college programs, at best, can be described as a survey course in nursing. The patient in the in-patient setting is not the focus of the curriculum of either educational program.

Again, this is significant because the in-patient setting constitutes the largest employer of nurses and remains the area of greatest need for nurses. In the 1980s, during a periodic surge in the chronic nursing shortage, the American Medical Association (AMA) introduced the concept of a registered care technologist. This proposed new job category would consist of individuals technically trained in many areas consistent with the competencies of the staff nurse. The proposal met with significant and effective opposition from the nursing establishment. However, the concept did not proceed into oblivion. It is still out there under such titles as healthcare technician and awaits its day in the sun. In the meantime, the nursing establishment appears impervious to the possibility of American nurses being supplanted by another type of patient care provider. In order to survive in the twenty-first century, a radically new approach to nursing education must emerge.

Improved image and social standing via attainment of professional status pervades many other issues in the evolution of American nursing. It is an intrinsic part of the story behind the participation of nurses in WWI and WWII. It is a major reason bedside hospital nurses made overtures to organized labor. It is the substance of the nursing establishment's demand for academic credentials as a prerequisite for nursing practice. It is intrinsic to the confusion caused by the existence of numerous nursing organizations and the failure of state boards of nursing to fulfill their mandate. This narrative examines the underlying dynamics of these issues. An example is found in Chapter 5, which deals with women activists of the early twentieth century who were part of the labor and suffrage movements. They are contrasted with the women of the nursing establishment. The latter were not involved with the labor movement; to have been would have been unprofessional. The nursing leadership assumed this stance while bedside nurses toiled away under difficult working conditions. The nursing leadership was a late supporter of women's right to vote. They feared alienating members of state government. The latter could impede passage of nurse licensing laws considered essential for recognition as professionals.

Probably many people outside academic nursing circles are not aware of the many reports on record from national committees, commissions, and forums addressing recurring issues within American nursing. The Carnegie Corporation, The Robert Wood Johnson Foundation, the Rockefeller Foundation, the Russell Sage Foundation, and the United States government all served as sponsors of appointed bodies that studied and issued reports on twentieth-century nursing. There is a specific instance where the nursing leadership publicly castigated recommendations put forth for their consideration. In 1970, recommendations were made by the National Commission for the Study of Nursing and Nursing Education in the Lysaught Report. The report made specific recommendations regarding the restructuring of nursing education. The nursing leadership of that era demonstrated a total disregard for the future of American nursing in their response to the recommendations of the Lysaught Report. Their response is examined in Chapter 11. Also in Chapter 11 is the author's proposal for the restructuring and renewal of nursing education in America.

This narrative is not a history of nursing, although the chapters do follow the historical timeline. There is a very brief historical synopsis of nursing in general. What follows is the agenda of influential American nurses of the nineteenth and early twentieth centuries and their efforts to influence the education of nurses. The narrative progresses through the Progressive Era, WWI and the Great Depression. These chapters describe lost opportunities.

The nursing leadership of that era rejected and/or ignored opportunities to alleviate the workplace hardships of the student and hospital nurse. The rationale for their behavior was always the advancement of nursing as a profession. During WWII nurses served on the home front, in the military, and initiated what would become a serious partnership with the American Labor Movement. Bedside nurses finally realized their concerns about working conditions and financial compensation were secondary to the foremost concern of twentieth-century nurse leaders—attainment of professional status.

Although not heard at the time, American nursing entered the second half of the twentieth century with a bang. A nurse functionary at Teachers College, Columbia University, initiated a two-year associate degree nursing educational program that changed the very character of American nursing. Very few in the nursing establishment identified the potential dangers associated with this new educational format to prepare students of nursing for the RN licensure examination. Most were preoccupied with the professional status and image issues.

The narrative proceeds with discussion of outstanding nursing issues of the latter part of the twentieth century. These include the ever-present nursing shortage, the quagmire created by numerous nursing organizations, legislative initiatives to mandate professional status via the baccalaureate degree, and nurse practitioners and primary nursing as final attempts at the professional dream. Also in the outstanding issue category is the 1965

American Nurses Association (ANA) Position Paper on Nursing Education. This manifesto insulted the majority of practicing nurses of that era and solidified the schism between academic nurses and worker nurses.

What is the root cause of the generalized incompetence of new graduate nurses? Is it legitimate or even ethical to sponsor educational programs that fail to provide students with the very basic skills needed for employment in the area of greatest need for nurses? What are the real factors supporting the chronic nursing shortage? How have some nursing leaders demonstrated an arrogance of leadership? How have state boards of nursing failed their mandate? What constitutes a durable nursing education program for the twenty-first century? The following chapters of this narrative provide some answers to these provocative questions and the answers are supported with documentation from American nursing's own literature.

2

IN THE BEGINNING

When God made man, he created nursing; ergo, nursing is as old as mankind. The mother feeding the child, the laying on of hands to soothe, and the bathing of the body to clean and render comfort are examples of nursing. The monitoring of a patient's heart rate, the changing of a patient's abdominal dressing, or teaching a diabetic patient to self-administer insulin are examples of nursing. Time changes many things, but the essence of nursing remains the same. Nursing means caring for another human being.

During the first half of the twentieth century, the history of nursing was a mandatory course for student nurses. The purpose was to impart an appreciation of the nursing tradition, and most students responded by memorizing names and dates. The majority of students simply wanted to get on to "real nursing." Eventually the nursing history course was eliminated from the basic nursing curriculum. Nursing educators explained that notable persons and significant historical events were now "integrated" into the total curriculum. This was a sign of the times. This was the new approach to teaching the sometimes dull tales of nursing history. Students should not be bored. Also the nursing establishment was emphasizing the image improvement plan. Certain historical facts, such as the domestic roots of nursing, did not support the image of the new professional nurse. Consequently, certain historical facts remained silent in the new integrated approach. Such accommodation was a mistake. The vocation of nursing lost a significant portion of its sense of self.

The traditional historical accounts of nursing start with ancient and early Christian civilizations, move through the Dark Ages, on to the Renaissance period to what is considered the modern period of nursing. This sequence demonstrates the omnipresence of nursing throughout the ages and the universal need for human beings to care for each other. Men as well as women provided nursing care, and both were frequently members of religious orders. Nursing was a calling or vocation to some individuals. To others, nursing was thrust upon them by the society in which they lived and many were not up to the challenge. These individuals, usually women, did what others refused to do or the religious were not available to do—care for the wretched sick poor who resided in alms-houses. Nightingale described these caregivers in the following manner.

> ...the women who embrace the office of nurse,
>   especially the Midwife for the poor, or of hospital

nurse, were generally those who were too old, too drunken, too dirty, too stolid, or too bad to do anything else. They were in fact, as nearly as possible, of the class from which now comes the "pauper nurse," for few women go into a workhouse except from defect, defect of some kind or other, defect of body, defect of mind, or defect of morality.(1)

The dual image of the nurse is apparent throughout the history of nursing: the God-fearing individual personified by members of religious organizations and the women described in the above quotation.

Eventually the need to educate the provider of nursing care was recognized. This is the beginning of the modern educational movement in nursing and is identified with the person of Theodor Fliedner (1800–1864). He established the Deaconess Institute at Kaiserswerth, Germany, in 1836; it consisted of a hospital and school for the training of deaconesses in the care of the sick.(2,3) In July 1861, the thirty-two-year-old Florence Nightingale (1820–1910) came to the Kaiserswerth Institute for three months of training and observation.(4) Nightingale was an interesting woman. She was well educated and well traveled. Her family held membership in the upper stratum of British society. She was presented at the court of Queen Victoria. It was unusual that a woman with this background would be interested in nursing. However, Nightingale was in search of a purpose. She viewed nursing as a calling, but in the secular sense. The catastrophe of war provided Nightingale the opportunity to realize her calling as a nurse.

The Crimean War (1853–1856) was fought between Russia and a coalition comprised of Great Britain, France, the Kingdom of Sardinia, and Turkey. Russia lost the war and Great Britain gained a heroine, the lady with a lamp. Nightingale took up the cause of the destitute wounded British soldier in the Crimea. It was his hell on earth. His basic human needs were not being met. In Scutari, he was housed in the large Barrack Hospital, lying in filth, vomit, and his own excrement. He was dying as a result of infected wounds, infestation of the environment, and inadequate medical and nursing care.

Fortunately, a British war correspondent, William Howard Russell, was reporting these conditions via a London newspaper. The British people became angry and demanded action. The Secretary of War, Sir Sidney Herbert, was aware the French wounded were receiving nursing care from the Sisters of Charity. He asked Nightingale to take a contingent of nurses to the Crimea.

Nightingale and thirty-eight nurses, many of them nuns, arrived in Scutari in November 1854. Nightingale found conditions as Russell had reported to the British public. She and her nurses were not welcomed by the medical establishment. These men were angry, unpleasant, and recalcitrant in their dealings with this independent woman. Regardless, Nightingale cleaned the Barrack Hospital and took care of the British soldier. Six months following her arrival the mortality rate was reduced from 42.7% to 2.2%.(5)

How was Nightingale able to have such an astounding impact on the welfare of these soldiers? She and her contingent of thirty-eight bathed the soldier, fed him, and provided him with a habitable environment. This was the work of nursing. Nightingale returned from the Crimea in 1856. Her accomplishments were recognized by the Queen and the British public. She was thirty-six years old and would live to be ninety. She remained involved in nursing affairs but never again engaged in direct nursing care.

Regardless of her limited exposure she deserves the title of founder of modern secular nursing. She earned this distinction by establishing, in 1860, a school of nursing at the St. Thomas Hospital in London. This was the first secular training program for nurses. The students had one year of formal training followed by two years of "experience." (This enforced experience of the Nightingale school is frequently ignored by American nurse historians. It was the same as the detested apprenticeship format that evolved in American hospital schools of nursing.) Nightingale was a perceptive and intelligent woman. She realized the care of the sick was moving into a different era, an era that could not accommodate the Sairey Gamps of the world. Previous to Nightingale's intervention, secular nursing was done by women with little training and likely with a shady past. It was not honorable to be a secular nurse in Victorian England. With Nightingale's influence, it became, at the very least, acceptable.

In Colonial America most nursing was done in the home. Only the homeless sick entered almshouses, not so much to be nursed but to die. The soldier of the Revolutionary War was cared for by camp followers. As usual, the religious nursing orders were a positive presence. They provided a high level of care to anyone who sought their assistance. Sometimes those who nursed were jail inmates who were sentenced to care for the sick. In New York, "ten-day women" were inmates from the workhouse on Blackwell's Island. They were sentenced to ten days, usually for public drunkenness. They would be released if they agreed to go to Bellevue Hospital and serve as a nurse for ten days.(6) Hospitals existed in this period of American history. The Pennsylvania Hospital was founded in 1752; the New York Hospital opened in 1791 and Massachusetts General Hospital opened in 1821.

It was difficult being a patient or caregiver in antebellum America. However some medical practitioners recognized the importance of providing those who nursed basic training that emphasized cleanliness of person and environment. They sought a woman who demonstrated a willingness to function under medical supervision. Joseph Warrington was a Quaker physician in Philadelphia. He was concerned about the quality of obstetrical care available to poor women. In 1839 he established the Nurse Society of Philadelphia. He trained nurses to go into the home and care for women during childbirth and the postpartum period.(7)

Dr. Elizabeth Blackwell (1821–1910) was the first woman in the United States to graduate from medical school. In 1857 she established the New York Infirmary for Women and Children and initiated a training program for nurses. Dr. Marie Zakrzewska (1829–1902) founded the New England Hospital For Women and Children in 1862. The act of incorporation identified the training of nurses as a major objective.(8) The importance of training nurses was recognized very early in American history and it was recognized primarily by physicians.

Although secular nursing in antebellum America received some enhancement, it remained essentially domestic in nature. This changed with the Civil War (1861–1865). In terms of nursing, it was America's Crimean War. There are many famous and noble women associated with this war. Clara Barton, Dorothea Lynde Dix, Mother Bickerdyke, The Woolsey sisters—Georgeanna Woolsey and Eliza Woolsey Howland—and Louisa Lee Schuyler. Collectively, the women of religious orders were again among the very first to volunteer as nurses. Author Louisa May Alcott rendered nursing care to the Union soldier and recorded her intense yet abbreviated experience as a Union nurse.(9)

The seminal idea on how to use the potential nursing skills of American women probably came from Blackwell. Blackwell was concerned about women rushing to the battlefield, void of any formal preparation in nursing. This was a valid concern. War was not a situation for zealous, idealistic, yet unprepared women. American women were well aware of the accomplishments of Nightingale and viewed this domestic crisis as an opportunity to follow in her footsteps.(10) At the outbreak of hostilities, the Union did not have a nurse corps, an ambulance service, field hospital system, or organized medical corps.(11) Blackwell took action. She proceeded to establish a month-long training course at Bellevue Hospital. Her objective was to prepare women to assume the duties of a wartime nurse. It is estimated that she prepared over one-hundred nurses for military service.(12) As a physician Blackwell understood the value of practical experience, and it is to her credit that she demanded experience at Bellevue for the would-be military nurses.

The transport women were an interesting group. They were atypical considering the era in which they lived. They were among the first female nurses to serve aboard a medical transport vessel. Many of these women were described as "displaced aristocrats."(13) The Woolsey sisters, Georgeanna and Eliza Howland, and Katherine Wormeley were such women. Together, during McClellan's Peninsular Campaign, they served on a river steamer. The steamers were utilized as an ambulance service. The sick and injured were removed from the Virginia peninsula and transported to northern hospitals. The Woolsey sisters had completed Blackwell's course at Bellevue.(14)

The United States Sanitary Commission (USSC) deserves mention. It played an important role in the Civil War and in the history of American nursing. The USSC was established by President Abraham Lincoln in June 1861. Prior to the Civil War, the government failed to make formal arrangements to care for the wounded soldier. The Army had a dismal record caring for those who fell in combat. They were frequently left to die on the battlefield. Now, in part through the auspices of the USSC, these matters were addressed.

The USSC was concerned with the health and sanitary needs of the Union soldier. Among its objectives was to supervise hospitals, recruit nurses and establish convalescent homes. For the first time in American history, female nurses would staff army hospitals. During the war years, USSC nurses and army contract nurses were an integral part of the military hospital system. The military, at the conclusion of the war, acknowledged the value of a properly trained nurse.

The oversight of army hospitals by the USSC had long-range implications for the American hospital system that emerged post Civil War. The Commission adhered to many of the principles put forth by Nightingale and incorporated many of those principles into hospital construction. For example, Nightingale advocated a facility that provided sunlight, fresh air, central heating, plumbing and laundry facilities, all under one roof.(15) The pavilion hospital met this criteria. The pavilion design was characterized by windows on both long sides of the ward, with doors at each end of the ward. The design called for a low, sprawling, one-story building.(16) The pavilion hospital became part of the American landscape. At the conclusion of the Civil War, the USSC had become the most powerful, most highly organized philanthropic activity in America.(17)

America did not have a Nightingale. The origins of modern American nursing were very "American." No one man or woman emerged as *the* leader of this new fledgling vocation for American women. Doctors, philanthropists, society women, and clergy all contributed ideas on how nurses and nursing could contribute to American society. There was no lady with a lamp in the American Civil War. There were many.

Secular nursing was evolving. The impetus for change was based in the social and scientific events that emerged in the nineteenth century. In his book *The History of Nursing*, Richard Shryock puts forth three explanations for the rise of modern secular nursing.(18) First, in both Great Britain and the United States, the origin is identified with the military services. The treatment and living conditions of the soldier in both wars were so deplorable, citizens demanded improved nursing services. Second is the spirit of humanitarianism, which he identifies as the driving force behind most social reforms of the era. An illustration of this concept is the women reformers of the nineteenth century and their impact on American nursing. This will be discussed in the next chapter. He identifies progress in the medical sciences as the third factor demanding improved nursing services. In the preface of the book, Shryock elaborates: "Within limits of available knowledge, moreover, the role of the nurse has often been conditioned by the role of the physician."

As medical knowledge expanded the physician took on new tasks and left the old tasks to the nurse. There was a time when a nurse was not allowed to measure blood pressure. Eventually the time arrived when the training of the nurse demanded the teaching of skills needed to do so. In her book *Nursing for the Future,* Esther Lucille Brown is quite specific regarding the relationship between physician and nurse. She operationally defined the relationship.

In clinical practice two distinct but interrelated kinds of functions have been most widely accepted as appropriate for the professional nurse to perform. One is the role of physician's assistant in carrying out technical procedures and treatments generally considered too complex or too dangerous to be entrusted to assistant personnel or to graduate nurses with only limited clinical training. The other is responsibility for critical observation of the patient, care of him sometimes for long periods without specific directions from the physician, and decision as to what should be reported, and when, to the doctor concerning the patient's condition.(19)

Brown's *Nursing for the Future* was written in 1948 and Shryock's *The History of Nursing* was written in 1959. Both authors were stating what was then considered obvious. Modern secular nursing was wedded to medicine and the advancement of medical knowledge. This was the nature of nursing. During the twentieth century the nursing establishment in America began to demonstrate an acceptance problem with these assumptions. The following chapters will discuss steps taken by the ladies of the establishment to forge an individual professional identity.

References

1. Seymer, Lucy R. *Selected Writings of Florence Nightingale.* New York: Macmillan Company. 1954. pg. 274.
2. Kalish, Philip and Kalish, Beatrice J. *The Advance of American Nursing.* Philadelphia: J.B. Lippincott Company. 1995 (3rd edition). pg. 28.
3. Donahue, Patricia M. *Nursing the Finest Art.* St. Louis: C.V. Mosby Company. 1985. pg. 234.
4. Dossey, Barbara Montgomery. *Florence Nightingale: Mystic, Visionary, Healer.* Pennsylvania: Springhouse Corporation. 1999. pg. 75.
5. Donahue. pg. 243–44.
6. Kalish and Kalish. pg. 64.
7. O'Brien, Patricia. "All a Women's Life Can Bring: The Domestic Roots of Nursing in Philadelphia, 1830–1885."

Nursing Research. January/February, 1987. Volume 36 #1. pg. 13.

8. Kalish and Kalish. pg. 67.

9. Alcott, Louisa May. *Hospital Sketches*. Reprint of 1863 edition. Chester Connecticut: Applewood Books. Distributed by Globe Pequot Press. 1993.

10. Giesberg, Judith Ann. *Civil War Sisterhood*. Boston: North Eastern Eastern University Press. 2000. pgs. 15–16.

11. Donahue. pg. 285.

12. Kalish and Kalish. pg. 63.

13. Garrison, Nancy S. *With Courage and Delicacy*. Mason City, Iowa: Savas Publishing Company. 1999. pg. 137.

14. Giesberg. pg. 119.

15. Garrison. pg. 4.

16. Rosenberg, Charles E. *The Care of Strangers*. New York: Basic Books. 1987. pg. 128.

17. Fredrickson, George M. *The Inner Civil War*. New York: Harper and Row. 1965. pg. 98.

18. Shryock, Richard. *The History of Nursing*. Philadelphia: W.B. Saunders Company. 1959. pg. 245.

19. Brown, Esther Lucille. *Nursing For the Future*. New York: Russell Sage Foundation. 1948. pg. 78.

3

ENTER LADY REFORMERS

"The Civil War, appalling calamity though it was, had two beneficent effects for American women. First, it raised nursing from a menial occupation to a dignified profession. Second, and more important, it taught women how to organize."(1)

The Civil War was a defining moment for American nursing. As in the Crimean War, the Nightingales of the Civil War made an important contribution, and history recognized that contribution. Furthermore, history recognized the contribution was made by the trained nurse, who, for the most part, was the product of the four-week course at Bellevue, first sponsored by Blackwell and later by the USSC.

The period immediately following the Civil War was described as "a wide open arena for women reformers."(2) There was a group of women who exerted considerable influence during the timeframe of post Civil War to the opening of the twentieth century. They are very important in telling the story of American nursing. They came primarily from the greater New York area and were members of influential families. These women were doers and contributors. They were concerned with the quality of hospital care in the United States. It was their belief that in order to reform the hospital situation, you must first reform nursing. They were the first in the United States to seriously approach the mission of reinventing the image of the nurse. They believed this was necessary in order to make nurses acceptable to physicians and to attract women of good character.

Louise Lee Schuyler (1837–1926) was a prominent member of this group. During the Civil War, Schuyler worked with Blackwell. Post Civil War, Schuyler turned her attention to many charitable and social endeavors. One day in the 1870s, Bellevue Hospital received a visit from a Committee of Ladies representing the New York State Charities Aid Association. The organization, the brain child of Schuyler, was comprised mostly of reform-minded society women. One of their most important activities was to monitor public hospitals.(3) The ladies found conditions at Bellevue far from satisfactory. They believed the right type of women could rectify the situation. Their remedy was the establishment of a school of nursing and the Bellevue Training School opened in May 1873.

The reform-minded society women assumed as did Nightingale that a woman of good character, from an acceptable family background, provided with theoretical and practical experience, could work near miracles.

Many of the Lady Visitors were veterans of the Civil War experience and they knew firsthand the positive impact of a trained nurse. Although they met with some resistance from the medical staff, the Lady Visitors persevered and made a dramatic point to Bellevue staff physicians.

Bellevue was experiencing a significant incidence of puerperal fever. This was an infectious disease sometimes called childbed fever. It could sweep through a ward and kill many new mothers. Failure to wash one's hands between patients was a major factor in the spread of this infection. Like Nightingale in the Crimea, the Ladies took action. They removed new and expectant mothers to a special maternity ward staffed by nurses from the Bellevue Training School. The situation and survival of the patients improved significantly. According to contemporary standards, this was accomplished by instituting some very basic measures.

The nurses of the Bellevue Training School enforced standards of personal hygiene for both themselves and the patient, maintained environmental cleanliness, and provided adequate ventilation of the patient care area. The nurse as ward overseer proved to be an essential component to the wellbeing of the patient. The Ladies made their point—a trained nurse made a difference.

This was a major step in the image improvement plan for the nineteenth century vocation of nursing. The society women who emerged during and following the Civil War as activists for hospital reform firmly believed proper selection and training of students would correct the deficiencies of patient care found in the American hospital system. Along the way they laid the foundation for modern American nursing. They recognized the need

to change the nursing image. They instituted this change
by elevating nursing to a trained status. Like Nightingale
in the post-Crimea era, they became advisors to nursing
and relinquished their role as participants. These women
rarely became nurses, yet they displayed a willingness
during wartime to join the military as nurses, trained or
otherwise. This was dramatically illustrated during the
Civil War, the Spanish American War, and WWI. Illogical
as it may seem, there is a romantic view of war. Elizabeth
Blackwell knew this and insisted on training women before
sending them on their mission.

Charles Rosenberg, in his book *The Care of Strangers,*
discussed the post-antebellum years and the role of the
nurse in the evolving hospital system. He discussed how
important the nurse was to the patients' immediate
physical environment and to the patients' general wellbeing.
He made an astute observation. "It is ironic that all these
arguments, so plausible in their mid-century context, were
to become increasingly inconsistent with the profession's
future aspirations."(4) There indeed was considerable irony,
as the twentieth century would demonstrate. Eventually
the importance of what the nurse did to and for the
patient would be minimized in favor of more academic
concerns.

Bellevue Hospital became a focal point in the
endeavors of the lady reformers. It would also become
a focal point in the history of American nursing. The
Bellevue Training School was the American version of the
Nightingale System of nursing education.

The Nightingale System refers to the organizational
format of the nursing school opened by Nightingale

at the St. Thomas Hospital in London. The school was financially independent of the hospital. This independence was the hallmark of the Nightingale System. The students were responsible to a head mistress and not to male physicians or board of directors. This was the Victorian Era. Nightingale wanted her school and students free of the male domination so characteristic of the times.

In contrast, under the Bellevue system in the United States, schools of nursing initially reported to committees or boards of lady overseers. Eventually the schools were absorbed into the hospital system, losing any separate and distinct identity. The integration of school into the hospital domain became the hallmark of the American system. Also, this integration would eventually become the source of great unrest among the evolving American nursing establishment.

There is another interesting aspect of Nightingale's belief system concerning training schools for nurses. The lady with the lamp distinguished between ordinary nurses and lady nurses. The former were not well educated and relied on a special school fund for expenses. The latter were considered gentlewomen, paid their own expenses, and expected to assume leadership positions at completion of the program.(5)

This raises an interesting question about Nightingale and her influence on American nursing. Did the founder of secular/modern nursing plant the seed for a strong emotional divide among nurses in the twentieth century? In American nursing, there are those who provide direct nursing care and those who teach nursing or direct others who provide the nursing care. Are those who provide direct nursing care the equivalent of the ordinary nurses as perceived by Nightingale? Are those who teach and direct those who provide nursing care the equivalent of the lady nurses? One must question if Nightingale's distinction became part of the thinking process, at least at the subconscious level, of members of the American nursing establishment. Keep in mind Nightingale's distinction between ordinary and lady nurses as decisions and actions of the nursing establishment are examined in future chapters.

The Bellevue Training School was one of three nursing schools to open in 1873. The Connecticut Training School was established at the New Haven State Hospital. Georgeanna Woolsey Bacon, of transport nurse fame, was a major player in the establishment of this school. The Boston Training School was established at Massachusetts General Hospital. The Women's Educational Association laid the groundwork for this school. The initial programs were two years in length, twelve-hour days and a half day off during the week. Student life was difficult. Students were responsible for domestic as well as nursing duties. They scrubbed floors as well as patients. By anyone's standards, the workload was overwhelming. They lived in simple if not stark living quarters that they could not leave without permission from some authority figure. Sara E. Parsons, an 1893 graduate of the Boston Training School at Massachusetts General Hospital, probably said it best.

The one outstanding error that has prevailed throughout the whole nursing system, and this School cannot be excepted, has been the assumption that overwork and severe discipline were necessary and even desirable concomitants of nurses in training. When it began to be understood that there was a difference between the self-imposed hardships and sacrifices of the religious orders and the preparation of modern young women for a profession, it was then impossible for economic reasons to lift the superfluous load that had broken the health of many good women during the early years of training schools, when only about fifty percent could or would stand the strain.(6)

So why did they do it? Why did women become student nurses? Why did they allow themselves to be utilized as a source of cheap labor? The economic depression of 1873, like the one that would occur in the twentieth century, answers part of the question why a young woman would want to become a student of nursing. The hospitals provided room, board, and a small stipend. Considering the times, these young women made a rational choice. As Richard Shryock points out in his history text, the conditions of work did not seem as difficult as they would today. Long hours with minimal pay were characteristic of farming, business, and industry. (7) Although these late nineteenth century women were decades away from voting rights, property rights, and legal access to birth control, they were beginning to seek independence. Some of these women came from middle-class homes and sought refuge from the tedium of a homebound existence. There were also those who found themselves without male financial support and realized they had to go it alone. However, in the post Civil War era, the majority of student nurses were not recruited from middle- or upper-class families.(8) In any case, they were all strong-willed women.

Linda Richards (1841–1930) deserves special mention. History texts identify Richards as the first trained nurse in the United States. Richards was awarded a nursing diploma from the New England Training School in 1873. This was another nursing school founded by a woman physician, Susan Dimock. Richards held many important positions, some with considerable name recognition. She was superintendent at two of the most famous schools of the United States, the schools at Bellevue and Massachusetts General Hospital. She helped establish the nursing school at Boston City Hospital. In 1886, she established the first training school for nurses in Japan. In her autobiography, *Reminiscences of Linda Richards,* she details many other positions.(9) She never stayed too long in any one assignment. One of her longest stays, five years, was at the school in Kyoto, Japan.

Richards was a doer. Surprisingly, nursing history texts do not demonstrate a great deal of interest in Richards's accomplishments. She is not considered part of the nursing elite. Perhaps this is because she spent more time "doing" nursing than "contemplating" nursing. Perhaps it stems from what she did when she helped establish the training school at Boston City Hospital. "Richards accepted, perhaps encouraged, the shift of nursing's line accountability to medicine from the Boards of Lady Managers when Boston City Hospital opened its training school with her as superintendent."(10) By agreeing to be organizationally accountable to medicine, Richards relinquished the hallmark of the Nightingale system—independence. Critics of Richards say she allowed medicine to dominate nursing. However, one nurse historian points out that nursing has always been dominated by an external force. In England, it was in the person of Nightingale, and in America, it was initially boards of philanthropic women.(11) Perhaps Richards was simply a pragmatic woman. This was America and in America the business aspects of a venture must be considered. The apprentice student nurse was an important financial asset to the hospital and as such should be an integral part of the system. The apprentice student nurse became the hallmark of the American system of nursing education and remained an integral part of the hospital system well into the twentieth century.

In 1907, Adelaide Nutting and Lavinia Dock authored a nursing history textbook. Utilizing a somewhat romantic frame of reference, they put the Civil War and immediate post-Civil War era into perspective. They wrote the following:

> The war came to an end, but the splendid work of the women on the Sanitary commission and of the nurses in the field could not die away. Their aroused energies could not be stifled, nor their fields of activity be again restricted. When they returned from military service it was to take up with moral courage and determination a new campaign for the reformation of civil institutions. The establishment of trained nursing in America came as the result of the war almost as directly as it had done in England.(12)

The genteel society ladies had successfully fashioned a new vocation for American women. As the new century approached, they departed the nursing scene and a very different type of nursing leader emerged. The new leaders were also concerned about improving the image of the nurse. However, the new leaders would approach the matter from a different perspective. The new leaders would seek a professional image for the twentieth century nurse.

References

1. Irwin, Inez Hayes. *Angels and Amazons.* New York: Doubleday, Doran and Company, Inc. 1933. pg. 150.
2. Ehrenreich, Barbara L. and Deirdre English. *Witches, Midwives and Nurses: A History of Women Healers.* London: Writers and Readers Publishing Cooperative. 1976. pg. 52.
3. Starr, Paul. *The Social Transformation of American Medicine.* New York: Basic Books, Inc. 1982. pg. 155.
4. Rosenberg, Charles. *The Care of Strangers.* New York: Basic Books, Inc. 1987. pg. 219.
5. Donahue, Patricia M. *Nursing the Finest Art.* St. Louis: C.V. Mosby Company. 1985. pg. 248.
6. Parsons, Sara E. *History of the Massachusetts General Hospital Training School for Nurses.* Boston: Whitcomb and Barrows. 1922. pg. 180.
7. Shryock, Richard. *The History of Nursing.* Philadelphia: W.B. Saunders Company. 1959. pg. 301.
8. Rosenberg. pg. 223.
9. Richards, Linda. *Reminiscences of Linda Richards.* Boston: Whitcomb and Barrows. 1911.

10. Baer, Ellen D. "Nursing's Divided House—An Historical View." *Nursing Research*. Volume 34. #1. (Jan/Feb) 1985. pg. 32.
11. *ibid*. pg. 36.
12. Nutting, Adelaide M. and Lavinia L. Dock. *A History of Nursing*. Volume 2. New York: G.P. Putnam and Sons. 1907. pg. 370.

4

GROUNDWORK FOR A BIG PROBLEM

American nursing has experienced many winters of discontent. The entire twentieth century was the one-hundred-year war with the hospital industry, with the medical establishment, and with self. The war with self was probably the most tragic. Early in the twentieth century, the nursing establishment, for understandable reasons, was troubled about society's image of the nurse. Professionalizing that image became their goal. The educational process became the vehicle of choice to reach that goal. An internal battle ensued regarding the correct form of nursing education. The nursing establishment became so consumed with the issue and the battle regarding nursing education that they neglected, ignored, or failed to recognize other important matters critical to American nursing. Perhaps the most critical oversight was the failure to recognize the incipient division within

American nursing. This oversight laid the groundwork for a big problem that would increasingly manifest itself throughout the twentieth century.

The genteel lady reformers of the post Civil War era brought needed changes to healthcare institutions. They established nurse training schools. They fostered a more positive image of those who would nurse for their livelihood. These ladies were a hard act to follow. In terms of a timeline, the professional status issue emerged with the immediate successors of the genteel lady reformers. These new major players in the story of American nursing were not from the privileged social class of their predecessors. These new leaders were from working-class families. Some had emigrated from Canada. These new leaders immediately focused on the goal of professional status for nurses. Why was this issue so important to these women? From their conscious perspective it was all about improving the image of nurses and nursing. They wanted to be viewed as women of good character and thus attract other women of good character to nursing. They undoubtedly sought some form of parity with the genteel image of their immediate predecessors. Regardless of their motivation, they were relentless in their pursuit of improved status for the nurse. Who were these women who laid the foundation for a tumultuous twentieth century for American nursing? Who was chief among this group destined to become the early nursing establishment? Teresa Christy, a nurse historian, identified three individuals as the most significant American nursing leaders of this era. They were Isabel Hampton-Robb, M. Adelaide Nutting, and Lavinia Loyd Dock.(1)

Isabel Hampton-Robb (1860–1910) was born in Welland, Ontario. Her early education prepared her to teach school, which she did for a period of three years. She departed Canada, entered Bellevue Training School for Nurses, and graduated in 1883. Historical accounts of Robb's early career place her in responsible positions soon after graduation. Before the age of thirty she was acting superintendent of nurses at Women's Hospital in New York and superintendent of nurses at the Illinois Training School. In 1889, she became the first leader of the new training school for nurses at John Hopkins Hospital. In this position, she demanded the title superintendent of nurses and principal of the Training School.(2)

The designation "principal" probably had special meaning for Robb. Like many early nursing leaders, Robb was a school teacher before she was a nurse, and she identified strongly with the role of educator. The role of educator would supersede her role as nurse. The teaching of nurses rather than the nursing of patients became the focal point of her nursing career. This was characteristic of many nursing leaders throughout the history of American nursing. Robb was a prominent member if not the lead member of the group agitating for professional status for nurses. She advocated for state regulation of nursing (licensure), generally viewed as a required step toward the attainment of professional status. Robb advanced two initiatives that contributed significantly to the inner chaos of American nursing throughout the twentieth century. Robb supported the formation of two nursing organizations, one for nurse educators and one for everyone else who nursed for a living. This was a major misjudgment on her part. She was the major influence in extending hospital diploma programs from two to three years. Both of these issues will be discussed in greater detail as the narrative proceeds. Robb's influence on American nursing was curtailed by her accidental death at the age of fifty.

M. Adelaide Nutting (1858–1948) was born in Quebec, Canada. Her formal education was directed primarily toward art and music. At age thirty-one, she became a member of the first class at John Hopkins Training School for Nurses. In 1907, she assumed a position at Teachers College, Columbia University. In 1910, she was awarded the title Professor of Nursing Education. Nutting was the first nurse to be appointed to a university professorship. (3) This was quite an accomplishment for a woman who did not have formal academic credentials. Nutting's nursing career was spent primarily in academic settings. Her major aspiration was to have basic training of nurses accomplished at the university level.

Lavinia Lloyd Dock (1858–1956) was born in Harrisburg, Pennsylvania. Nurse historians describe her as well educated and refer to her accomplishments as an organist and pianist. Dock graduated from Bellevue Training School for Nurses in 1886. She held numerous nursing positions, usually of short duration. She was superintendent of nurses at the Illinois Training School. Of this experience she said, "I was a perfect failure." (4) Dock worked with Lillian Wald at the Henry Street Settlement. Dock was a writer. She wrote a textbook about drugs and solutions titled *Materia Medica for Nurses*. She authored or co-authored a number of nursing history texts. She identified male domination of the health field as the source for all that plagued the nurse and nursing.(5) She was probably one of the first to go on record with these concerns. She went to jail three times in support of women's suffrage.

Each of these individuals, Robb, Nutting, and Dock, represents a recurring theme in the story of American nursing. Robb represents the call for professional status. Nutting represents the call to academia. Dock represents the call to overthrow the forces that oppress nurses— specifically male physicians and hospital administrators.

Two nursing organizations were formed during the last decade of the nineteenth century. Robb, Nutting, and Dock were involved with the formation, but Robb was the primary moving force. The American Society of Superintendents of Training Schools for Nurses was founded in 1893. Membership was restricted to nurse educators. This organization was concerned with admission requirements and educational standards for training schools. To control admission requirements and educational standards was to control the type of women permitted membership to the fledgling would-be profession of nursing. The second organization, the Nurses' Associated Alumnae of the United States and Canada, was founded in 1897. The organization's primary goal was legal recognition of nursing in all states via registration and licensure. This was the organization for the rank and file. (6) The American Society of Superintendents of Training Schools for Nurses would become the National league of Nursing (NLN). The Nurses' Associated Alumnae of the

United States and Canada would become the American Nurses Association (ANA). These turn-of-the-century nursing leaders created an untenable situation by creating the two nursing organizations. These women, the seminal nursing establishment, essentially divided American nursing into two groups. Consequently, American nursing would never realize the potential to marshal forces, become a critical mass and speak with one voice.

> The decade of the 1890s had seen professionalization advance from little more than an idea in Isabel Hampton's head to seeming completion. And yet as the decade and the century ended, a feeling of frustration set in among the superintendents, as if the goal had somehow eluded their grasp.(7)

Indeed, the goal of professionalization had eluded these early leaders and would continue to do so for future generations of nurses.

Following the Civil War, hospital training programs for nurses emerged as two-year programs. Robb advocated the extension of the hospital training programs to three years. She gave the following explanation.

> ...a third year is to be regarded as a period of assimilation or digestion, without which the learning of the first two years will be far less valuable. That many nurses feel that they are not fully qualified at the end of two years is evidenced by the number of intelligent women who love their work and who are interested in their profession and who beg to be allowed to stay another year.(8)

Robb's explanation falls short of reality. The skill and knowledge base necessary for a nurse at the start of the twentieth century did not require an additional year of study or training. The country was recovering from a serious economic depression. Perhaps the students begging to stay on for a third year appreciated the room, board, and small stipend that came with student nurse status. Perhaps Robb wanted to emulate the Nightingale schools that required a third apprenticeship year for completion of the course of study. More likely Robb viewed the additional year as a means to the professional end. Robb was an advocate of the eight-hour day for the student nurse. It was difficult to attract the right type of woman to a twelve-hour workday. There could be a trade off with the hospital hierarchy. The deal would be an eight-hour work day for three years of apprenticeship training. No self-respecting hospital administrator could refuse Robb's proposal. Viewed from his perspective, this was an additional year of free labor. The deal was made, and thus the origin of the three-year hospital nurse training program in the United States. Robb was an idealistic Victorian woman, well meaning and naïve. Her naivete is displayed in the following statement.

> Many hospitals have adopted with readiness the third year, but only here and there, in very few schools indeed, have the hours in the wards been reduced to eight practical hours of work.(9)

Apparently Robb was not sophisticated in the ways of the new hospital industry. Apparently she did not appreciate the relationship between the economics of healthcare delivery in the hospital system and free services provided by young women known as student nurses.

The third year of the hospital training program was the brainchild of a prominent female nursing leader—not a male hospital administrator. The implementation of Robb's proposal would haunt nursing and nurse educators for the better part of the twentieth century. The three-year hospital training program would become, for nurse educators of the twentieth century, the essence of everything evil with nursing education. In 1922, twelve years following Robb's death, Nutting addressed the issue of the third year.

> Those of us who, many years ago, lengthened the two year course of training to three years, confident that this measure would solve many of the educational problems we were then struggling with, must surely see that we have not been able, even with our best efforts, to make the three years what we intended it should be educationally. We have found no just and certain way of utilizing for the benefit of our students, the full time of the added year.(10)

Holding steadfast to the image and professional status issue, Robb made yet another proposal affecting the wellbeing of the student nurse. This proposal concerned the stipend issue. Hospitals gave student nurses small monthly stipends. For some in the nursing establishment the stipend was viewed as payment for services rendered. Such payment was not consistent with a professional education. The payment was not consistent with the "right type of woman" scenario. The right type of woman would not need a stipend. Robb addressed the issue.

> It has been conceded that the old-time method of giving a monthly allowance to each pupil was to be deplored on the principle that it lessened the educational value of the instruction and that it was far better to give an education commensurate for services rendered.(11)

Hospital administrators were not eager to implement Robb's stipend elimination proposal. To them it was not a moral issue but a common sense issue. Student nurses were working twelve-hour days. If they had to work extra for spending money, they would get sick and leave the program. Stipends remained a practice well into the twentieth century. Early hospital administrators were callous with the time and lives of student nurses. However, the early nursing establishment also displayed a cavalier attitude regarding the time and lives of student nurses. What was one more year of apprenticeship from a young woman's life? What were a few dollars to a young woman's wellbeing? After all, it was for a good cause—the professionalization of nursing.

In 1890, there were thirty-five schools of nursing in the United States. In 1900, there were 432 schools.(12) The proliferation of schools of nursing corresponded to the proliferation of hospitals. Hospitals of all sizes had schools of nursing. They were an integral part of large teaching hospitals such as Hopkins or Bellevue. They were an integral part of fifty-bed rural hospitals.

The hospital training program was an apprenticeship system. The training of the student nurse was secondary to the provision of nursing care to patients. Student nurses were the lifeblood of the hospital. They were economic assets. They provided a continuous service to patients. They worked all day, every day with minimal time off. They were a source of income. Students were sent into homes for private duty, and their fee for services rendered was paid directly to the hospital. Nursing students were an inexpensive, stable, and disciplined workforce.(13) Nursing students, the primary nursing staff of the hospital, kept hospital costs artificially low. This fact eventually created a serious economic problem for the evolving American hospital system.(14) (During the timeframe under discussion, graduate nurses were not employed as staff nurses in hospitals. Staff nurses were a later phenomena of the twentieth century.)

The three-year hospital training program lasted well into the mid-twentieth century before declining in significant numbers. The reasons for the decline were twofold. Young women turned to the college setting for their post high school education. Secondly, hospital training programs became too expensive to operate. Accrediting bodies such as the National League of Nursing and State Boards of Nursing demanded hospitals stop utilizing student nurses as an integral part of their workforce. They demanded students be treated as students. Eight-hour days and five-day work weeks became part of the price for program accreditation and/or state approval for operation of a training program.

By the mid-1950s hospital training programs became less attractive to both potential students and hospital administrators. Interestingly, in 1911, the California State Legislature passed a law limiting the hours a woman could work. The law did not include hospitals. In 1913, the California labor movement successfully pressured the Legislature to include student nurses in the provisions of the law.(15) The first relief for student nurses came from the efforts of the labor movement, not state boards of nursing, educational accrediting organizations, or the nursing establishment. The latter would remain aloof from the labor movement for *professional* reasons. This will be discussed in greater detail in the next chapter.

Robb and Nutting continued their crusade to professionalize nursing. Image enhancement of American nursing would now be attempted via the academic route. Their quest brought them to Teachers College, Columbia University. Again, Robb had an idea. She wanted nurses to have entrée into the college setting. She approached Dean James Earl Russell for the purpose of establishing a course in hospital economics.(16) Russell agreed with Robb's proposal, and the initial course was offered in 1899. The course would be geared toward nurse educators and superintendents of nurses. This was the first formal collegiate program of study for nurses.(17) Thus began American nursing's long association with Teachers College and the academic world. The marriage of nursing and academia would have far reaching effects.

The nursing leaders of this era did not grasp the total picture in terms of American society's expectations of nursing. They either failed to realize or simply ignored the fact there was lack of public support for their self-prescribed mission to professionalize the vocation of nursing. Also, they either failed to realize or simply ignored the fact there was ample support among the public for the training of nurses via the hospital apprenticeship system. At the turn of the twentieth century both the hospital and the public benefited from this system: "…apprenticeship was a cheap plan requiring no public support from a monetary standpoint."(18) As far as the general public was concerned, the hospitals were providing the students with a good deal.

There were other problems caused by the leaders' failure to recognize certain realities of the day. They were not providing the leadership necessary to influence day-to-day operations of hospital training programs that impacted so greatly on the student nurse's life. The leaders did not display a sense of urgency in resolving the practical problems of the student nurse in the work situation. They failed to seek the assistance of the labor movement in resolving these problems. They ignored the successful intervention of the California labor movement in 1913. Instead the leadership directed their energies to defining educational standards, improving the image of nurses and the ultimate in exclusionary tactics, seeking the registration and licensure of nurses. Eventually the fledgling nursing establishment sought a new platform from which to direct their energies in denouncing the hospital apprenticeship system for the training of nurses. They abandoned the hospital scene and transferred their energies and presence to the academic setting.

The two nursing organizations formed in the late nineteenth century evolved into two segments of American nurses. The nursing establishment in the persons of nursing educators and nursing superintendents represented one segment. The larger segment was represented by the nurse at the patient's bedside. By the early 1920s, the groundwork for the great divide in nursing was firmly established causing major and perhaps irreversible problems for American nursing throughout the twentieth century. And the groundwork was laid with a false premise: that nursing was a profession. The professional status issue became dogma and consumed the energy and common sense of many in nursing. As the new millennium approached the issue lost relevance for everyone except the members of the nursing establishment.

Abraham Flexner was a contemporary of Robb, Nutting, and Dock. He was a well-known American educator. He is best known for a report he wrote for the Carnegie Foundation. The report, *Medical Education in the United States and Canada*, also known as the Flexner Report, is considered by some to be responsible for significant reforms in the nation's medical schools. As the twentieth century advanced, the nursing establishment attempted to link numerous reports about needed reforms in American nursing to the Flexner Report. However, the nursing reports never achieved the level of impact or renown demonstrated by the Flexner Report. In 1915 Flexner presented a paper titled, *Is Social Work a Profession?* at the National Conference of Charities and Correction.

Apparently the social workers asked his opinion regarding the professional status of nurses. He made the following comment.

> The trained nurse is making a praiseworthy and important effort to improve the status of her vocation. She urges, and with justice, that her position is one of great responsibility; that she possess knowledge, skill and power of judgment; that the chances of securing these qualifications, all of them essentially intellectual, improve, as the occupation increases in dignity. It is to be observed, however, that the responsibility of the trained nurse is neither original or final. She, too, may be described as another arm to the physician or surgeon.(19)

History indicates the nursing establishment listened to Flexner, but apparently in a very selective manner. No one in nursing asked for clarification regarding his remarks to the social workers.

References

1. Christy, Teresa. "Portrait of a Leader: Lavinia Loyd Dock." *Nursing Outlook.* June 1969. pg. 73.
2. Christy, Teresa. "Portrait of a Leader: Isabel Hampton-Robb." *Nursing Outlook.* March 1969. pg. 27.
3. Christy, Teresa. "Portrait of a Leader: M. Adelaide Nutting." *Nursing Outlook.* January 1969. pg. 21.
4. As quoted in "Portrait of a Leader: Lavinia Dock." pg. 73.
5. Donahue, Patricia M. *Nursing the Finest Art.* St. Louis: C.V. Mosby Company. 1985. pg. 356.
6. *ibid.* pg. 361.

7. James, Janet Wilson. "Isabel Hampton and the Professionalization of Nursing" in *The Therapeutic Revolution*. Morris J. Vogel and Charles F. Rosenberg, editors. Philadelphia: University of Pennsylvania Press, 1979. pg. 234.

8. Birnbach, Netti and Sandra Lewenson, editors. *First Words: Selected Adresses from the NLN 1894–1933*. New York: National League for Nursing Press. 1991. pg. 16.

9. Robb, Isabel Hampton. "The Affiliation of Training Schools for Nurses for Educational Purposes." *American Journal of Nursing*. July 1905. pg. 668.

10. Nutting, M. Adelaide. *A Sound Basis for Schools of Nursing and Other Addresses*. New York: Garland Publishing Inc. 1984. pg. 288–90.

11. Robb. pg. 69.

12. Roberts, Mary M. *American Nursing*. New York: The Macmillan Company. 1954. pg. 5.

13. Rosenberg, Charles. *The Care of Strangers*. New York: Basic Books. 1987. pg. 220.

14. Ashley, JoAnn. *Hospitals, Paternalism and the Role of the Nurse*. New York: Teachers College Press. 1979. pg. 19.

15. IBID. pg. 40–41.

16. Christy, Teresa. "Portrait of a Leader: Isabel Hampton-Robb." pg. 28.

17. Hanson, Kathleen. "The Emergence of Liberal Education in Nursing." *Journal of Professional Nursing*. Volume 5 #2. March/April 1989. pg. 89.

18. Wolf, Karen. editor. *JoAnn Ashley: Selected Readings*. New York: National league for Nursing Press. 1997. pg. 223.

19. Flexner, Abraham. *Is Social Work a Profession?* New York: The New School of Philanthropy. 1915. pg. 4.

5

IN CONTEXT

The place is America. The timeframe is the Depression of the 1890s to the conclusion of World War 1. It was a time of social change and political ferment caused by industrialization, urban growth and ethnic tension.(1) It was a time of reform. It was the Progressive Era in American history. The influx of immigrants increased the populations of the cities, particularly on the eastern seaboard. The tenements of New York and Boston epitomized the congested, disease-ridden sanctuaries called home by poor Americans or would-be Americans.

It was the era of the "muckrakers," the term coined by Teddy Roosevelt to describe investigative reporters who exposed corruption and scandal in politics and industry.(2) One such muckraker was a woman, Ida Tarbell. She authored an investigative piece titled, "History of the Standard Oil Company," an exposé of the

Rockefeller Corporations. She described the corruption of governments, extortion of privileges and crushing of competition.(3) Tarbell's work was influential in the breakup of the Standard Oil Company of New Jersey in accordance with the 1911 Sherman Anti-Trust Act.

Dorothy and Carl Schneider, in their work *American Women in the Progressive Era, 1900–1920,* described it best when they wrote, "In 1900 all these American women were living in difficult as well as interesting times, changing times." (4) This was the era of the suffrage movement, the early feminist movement, the demand for legal access to birth control, and the uprising of the female garment workers. It was a time when some women of America demanded to be part of the dynamics of reform. Not all women took up the banner, but those who did were very interesting people. They were socialists, communists, and anarchists. Some were lesbians. Others were socialites, actresses and factory workers. Some were college graduates. Others had a high school diploma, and others did not go past the eighth grade. They were as different as night and day. The one thing they had in common was the belief that women deserved a better deal.

A better deal for women could not be had without the right to vote. The suffrage movement for American women began in 1848 at the Women's Rights Convention in Seneca Falls, New York and was successfully concluded in 1920 by ratification of the Nineteenth Amendment. The suffragettes fought hard for the franchise. They experienced assaults by hoodlums and the humiliation of imprisonment with threats of forced feedings.(5)

The fight pitted them against men and other women.
The prospect of women as a voting block scared the
bejesus out of many a man of the day. It took a long time,
but the women persevered. Not all suffragettes were
feminists. The suffragettes can be considered conservative
in outlook when compared to feminists. Feminists
demanded more than the right to vote. To feminists,
obtaining the right to vote was just a step in the right
direction. In her book, *To Be Young Was Very Heaven*, Sandra
Adickes elaborates in detail about the Progressive Era
feminist. She writes women who defined themselves as
feminists were "advocates of radical trends and behavior
in the labor movement, art and politics." She describes the
feminists as standing for "self-development rather than self-
sacrifice or submergence in the family."

Feminists wanted the right to work; the right to be a
mother and work in a profession; the right to keep her
own surname and the right to organize.(6) These were
stunning demands for the times, and immediate attainment
was not in the cards. However, the feminists of the
Progressive Era set the stage for the women who assumed
the cause in later decades of the twentieth century.

There was the matter of birth control. Women of
this era, particularly poor women, uneducated women,
and immigrant women, did not have information or legal
access to birth-control measures. There were major
factors working against women who wanted control of
their reproductive functions. One such factor was the
Federal Comstock Laws, a series of anti-birth-control
laws. Another factor was fear regarding the influx of Asian

immigrants. This fear was coupled with "race suicide" anxiety. This was code for the threat to the white race posed by women who desired fewer children and smaller families. And of course there was the Catholic Church.(7)

However, there was also an individual who stepped forward and advocated for the right of women to have information about and access to birth-control measures. Her name was Margaret Sanger (1883–1966). Sanger, a nurse, graduated from White Plains Hospital, located near New York City. Her nursing experience consisted of public health nursing in New York's Lower East Side. She witnessed the tragedies of mothers who did not know how to prevent an unwanted pregnancy. They begged Sanger to tell them the secrets of the rich women. Sanger left nursing and concentrated on the dissemination of birth-control information. She became an activist in this regard and spent time in jail for the cause.

The Progressive Era witnessed the tragedy of the Triangle Shirtwaist Fire and the uprising of female garment workers. Between 1909 and 1915, thousands of garment workers in the Northeast and Midwestern states called strikes, demanding better working conditions and recognition of their unions.(8) It was the era of concerned middle class women taking an interest in the working conditions of young female workers. These women were instrumental in establishing Working Girls Clubs, YWCAs and passage of protective legislation for women in the work place.(9)

How did a career as a nurse fit into the Progressive Era? It fell far short of the professional aspirations of the leadership. There was not even the façade of professional status for most nurses. Nurses had three options for employment. If she graduated from one of the elite schools such as Bellevue or Hopkins, she might be offered a position in the hospital setting as a supervisor or teacher of nurses. The second option was employment as a public health nurse. The growth of cities, the phenomenal rise of industry and the influx of an immigrant population gave rise to conditions that imperiled many people. The tenement enclaves harbored tuberculosis and other life-threatening communicable diseases. Infant mortality, maternal morbidity and mortality gave rise to an appalling atmosphere for any social-minded health-oriented person. Enter the public health nurse, teacher of health promotion and disease prevention. This was definitely her era.

The nursing establishment perceived the public health nurse as one of their own—a real professional nurse. Part of this perception had to do with the public health nurse's seemingly independent operational work style. A great deal of the nurse's workday was spent teaching patients rather than providing direct nursing care. This teaching activity, accompanied by an unstructured and relatively unsupervised work environment, reinforced her elevated status among other nurses. Her relationship with patients was quite different from that of other nurses. It was intermittent rather than continuous, resembling the physician-patient relationship. Lay women directed many of the agencies that employed public health nurses. This placed the nurses out of the reach and control of physicians and hospital administrators. She usually had post-graduate education. All these characteristics supported the professional image, so important to the nursing establishment.

There was an aura of adventure and idealism surrounding public health nurses. They commanded respect as they made their rounds in their tailored uniforms, prim hats, carrying their little black bags. They were worshiped by and had the eternal gratitude of their patients. They in turn worshipped Lillian D. Wald and Mary Brewster, who founded the Henry Street Visiting Nurse Service, the House on Henry Street. Many of these women, like Lavinia Dock, were social and political activists. Public health nurses became an elite corps within nursing.(10)

However, the needs of American society changed. Karen Buhler-Wilkerson points out by the late 1920s, public health nursing had reached a turning point. They were assuming an increasingly marginal role in the healthcare system. There was significantly less immigration, growing emphasis on the hospital as a refuge for the sick, and the declining impact of infectious disease.(11) The work and mission of the public health nurse gradually went into obscurity.

The remaining option for a new graduate nurse and the most common was private duty nursing. In nursing circles, the nurse educator was highest in status, followed by the poster child of the era, the public health nurse. The private duty nurse, the direct caregiver, was low person on the totem pole. Initially, private duty nursing meant caring for a patient in the home. The private duty nurse found a patient, "her case," through a variety of mechanisms such as word of mouth, referrals from physicians, patients, pharmacists, and nurse registries.(12) There was nothing really attractive about her life. Some would say she was free and independent but in reality she required the help of a number of people to maintain regular employment. According to arrangements she made with the family, her tour of duty could be twelve or twenty-four hours. Depending on the social status of the family, her status within the household could resemble that of domestic help. The private duty nurse lived an isolated existence. Her work was solitary. She did not have the companionship of colleague nurses. Due to time constraints, personal interests were denied an outlet.

By the mid-1920s, the number of sick people cared for in the home diminished considerably. They were now going into the hospital. They had hospital insurance plans. Physicians were in favor of hospitalization because of the need for fewer house calls. Newer treatment modalities were suited only for the hospital setting. The private duty nurse reluctantly went into the hospital with her patient. However her social and professional isolation remained intact. She cared for only one patient among many, and this was a source of irritation to student nurses who cared for all others. Her access to in-service education was limited, providing an image of an individual out of touch with real nursing. In 1929, the Great Depression shattered the world of the private duty nurse. The patient could no longer afford her services. The Great Depression ended the dominance of the private duty nurse as the largest segment of American nurses.

What can be said of the American nursing establishment in terms of the Progressive Era? How did they view the message of reform so intrinsic to this segment of American history? Some consider nurses to be the most conservative of the conservative. One nurse historian attributes this conservatism to the failure of the nursing establishment to "liberate" nursing.(13)

For the purposes of this narrative, the nursing establishment will be assessed in terms of involvement or lack of involvement, in three specific areas: the suffrage issue, the labor movement, and licensure of nurses. Of the first, the suffrage issue, the leadership in general tried to ignore, avoid but eventually dealt with the issues in a marginal manner. The second, the labor movement, was considered an anathema to be avoided at all costs. In terms of licensure, the nursing establishment partially achieved their goals.

Most nurses were late advocates of suffrage for American women. The suffrage movement in the U.S. began in 1848. It was 1912 before organized nursing officially endorsed the movement, just eight years before the amendment was ratified.

Lavinia Dock was one of the few nurses who did not fit the mold. In Chapter 4, Dock was described as a feminist and an intellectual. She was atypical. Most of her nurse contemporaries were not intellectuals or feminists. In 1907, Dock addressed the Nurses Alumnae Association. The address was titled, "Some Urgent Social Claims." She encouraged her audience to look beyond their immediate sphere and place nursing in a broader context. Dock was referring specifically to women's suffrage. In part, she said the following:

I would like to see our national body leave all smaller concerns to the local societies and consciously make itself a moral force on all the great social questions of the day, and I would like to have our journals not afraid to mention the words political equality for women.(14)

Dock's reference to journals was probably specific to the *American Journal of Nursing* (AJN). The AJN maintained a neutral stance on the suffrage issue. This neutrality changed to support in 1913, following the ANA's endorsement. Dock remained quite public in her advocacy and used the column she wrote for the AJN to publicize that support. Dock was certainly not the only nurse to support suffrage, but she was certainly the most visible. Eventually Dock, like Sanger, left nursing and devoted her time and efforts to broader social issues.

One can speculate that both women activists found the conservatism of American nursing too overbearing in this age of reform. An important question remains to be answered. Why was the nursing establishment so tardy in rendering official support for the suffrage movement? Sandra Beth Lewenson discusses this issue in her book *Taking Charge, Nursing Suffrage and Feminism in America 1873–1920*. There was the licensing issue. This could only be implemented by state legislatures. Lewenson speculates there was reluctance to pursue the suffrage issue due to fear of alienating the male legislator. Also, the nursing establishment was busy pursuing more mundane matters such as preferred character traits for nursing school applicants and the issue of nursing programs being two or three years in length, etc. The practicing nurse did not advocate for suffrage because she was fearful of losing her livelihood. Their work situation was described as "an often hostile, conservative male dominated work environment."(15)

However, nurses eventually supported suffrage. Their delay in standing up to be counted, particularly in the Progressive Era, is noteworthy. They were conservative by nature, insecure, afraid, and parochial. These are not characteristics of risk takers. Also, these very characteristics coupled with the dominance of the professional issue likely contributed to the failure of nurses to embrace the labor movement at this juncture in their history.

In 1913 Lavinia Dock made her final speech to a nurses' convention. The title of the speech was "Status of the Nurse in the Working World."(16) Dock addressed the issue of nurses and the labor movement. She made a rather astounding statement. She said the following:

> That the nurse is a worker no one can deny. However high professionally she may build her career, however distinguished and noble she may make it, and we all feel, thankfully, that the nature of our work sets no limits in these directions, she is still closely related to the world of workers whom we call toilers.

There was no pretense about being a professional. Nurses were toilers. They were workers. She went on to tell the same audience that the hours workers must sustain to earn a livelihood should be of paramount importance to nurses. Dock implies the nursing organization had formally ignored the hours of work issue because of fear of being identified with "trade unionism." Again, in the same speech Dock describes a situation in Massachusetts. Apparently there was proposed legislation aimed at controlling the number of hours an individual could work. Dock described doctors and nurses appearing before the state legislature to address the issue. According to Dock, they implored the legislature not to pass a law fixing hours of work. According to Dock, the doctors and nurses believed such a law would injure their professional honor. More likely they simply feared association with anything "union like."

During the Progressive Era there were two categories of nurses working excessive number of hours. They were the private duty nurse and the nursing student. The nursing establishment did very little on behalf of either group. The private duty nurse was very much a part of her own problem. It has been pointed out "by circumstance and by tradition, the private duty nurse was an individualist and a loner." The private duty nurse represented the largest segment of nurses yet kept her distance and her clout from nursing organizations, specifically the ANA.(17) The loner is not a joiner. Also, the nursing establishment was really not interested in her plight. Their primary focus was the making of a profession. In return, the ideology and strategies of the nursing establishment were viewed by the private duty nurse as irrelevant.(18) The nursing establishment had little to offer the private duty nurse. Their response to the trials and tribulations of the largest segment of practicing nurses of that era was to espouse higher standards of admission to nursing schools. The rationale was that the higher standards would help decrease the production of graduate nurses. This in turn would lessen the competition for the private duty nurse. The private duty nurse, a direct caregiver, represented a conflict of interest for the image sensitive nursing establishment. These direct caregivers represented the domestic roots of nursing.

Student nurses worked an excessive number of hours, and this fact is well documented. Sixteen hours a day and six-and-one-half days per week were the usual. These long hours remained a reality for student nurses long after female garment workers gained relief from their long workdays. The nursing establishment of this era bemoaned the plight of student nurses. Their concerns are well documented in nursing journals and in testimony to investigative groups looking into the "nursing situation." However, they did little else about the situation except blame hospital administrators.

Hospital administrators were indeed at fault. They had a great deal of control over the daily activities of student nurses and they exercised that control. The nursing establishment was also at fault. They did not challenge hospital administrators. However, what could they do—call a strike? Professionals do not strike. One can speculate what would have happened if the nursing establishment discarded the pretense of pseudo-professionalism and sought the assistance of their more progressive sisters in the labor movement. Well, it did not happen, and the life of the student nurse remained dismal well into the twentieth century. The nursing establishment did not want to associate with the labor movement. To compensate and on behalf of the student nurse, they created the persona of victim. This persona remains with American nurses to this day.

Clinging to the illusion of professionalism caused other serious problems for American nursing. It impeded the organizing of nurses into a functioning whole. The nursing establishment of this era consisted mainly of nurse educators and nursing superintendents. Their numbers were few in comparison to direct caregivers, the people Dock called "toilers." The first group was concerned about status. The second group was concerned about bread-and-butter issues. This difference in focus kept the elites and toilers from becoming a cohesive group of nurses with influence that could make a difference. Consequently, American nursing was not taken seriously as a social or political force. This was true during the Progressive Era and remains true today.

The goal of licensure was a partial success for the nursing establishment. In the time frame of 1900–1920, the acquisition of licensing laws dominated the political agenda of nursing.(19) In the early twentieth century, the licensing of individuals to work in a specific occupation was a crucial step in obtaining professional status for members of that occupation. Teachers, social workers, and nurses all sought professional recognition via licensure. The motivating factors were status, economics and the control of education of would be practitioners.(20) In terms of the latter, the state imposes regulations concerning minimum admission criteria and minimum standards for curriculum of professional educational programs. There are important secondary effects resulting from these regulations such as the exclusionary effect. An example was the action taken by the State of New York regarding admission requirements to schools of nursing. In 1906, the State mandated that students entering schools of nursing were required to have at least one year of high school education.(21) This definitely narrowed the applicant field. Not everyone went to high school in the early years of the twentieth century.

The state mandated minimum curriculum requirements. Many nursing schools did not offer a course in obstetrical nursing. Once the state identified obstetrical nursing as a minimum requirement, schools were required to provide course work and clinical experience in obstetrical nursing. This required smaller or specialized hospitals to either close their school or establish an obstetrical affiliation with another institution.

Needless to say there was strong opposition to many of these new regulations. Hospital administrators offered major opposition. From their perspective mandated admission requirements decreased the size of the applicant pool and affiliations cost money. However they complied; it was the law.

State imposed curriculum requirements also impacted atypical schools of nursing. An example of an atypical school was the Chautauqua School of Nursing which, via mail, "trained women in their own home to earn $12 to $30 per week."(22) Before the existence of licensing laws, a piece of paper from one of these "schools" allowed an individual to present herself as a trained nurse and remain within the confines of the law. Many individuals did just that. This contributed to the poor public image of nurses and definitely maximized the numbers of individuals seeking positions as private duty nurses.

The nursing establishment viewed licensing laws as the answer to their major obstacle, their lack of control of the education of nurses. With these laws they would control the education and the destiny of nursing, or so they thought. These laws, administered by state boards of nursing, had significant potential to positively impact American nursing. However, as the twentieth century advanced, state boards of nursing failed to realize this potential. Instead, state boards of nursing made significant contributions to the internal chaos of American nursing.

The first nurse licensure law was enacted in 1903 by the State of North Carolina. In the same year New Jersey, New York, and Virginia enacted similar laws. There was a flaw in these laws. They were permissive, not mandatory. Practice of nursing was not limited to persons licensed by the state. Unlicensed persons could still represent themselves as a nurse. What they could not do is represent themselves as a registered nurse. It would be mid-century before this situation was corrected.

Tomes believes nurse historians minimized the degree of opposition to these laws and perpetuated the belief licensing laws achieved the goals espoused by the nursing establishment.(23) Opposition was to be expected. Enactment of laws means politics and politics means special interests. Physicians saw licensing as a power play on the part of nurses. They viewed nurses as attempting to gain parity with physicians via the licensing route. Hospital administrators certainly did not want the state telling them how to operate their schools. The home-grown nurse feared loss of livelihood. Of course, these special interest groups and many others like them either opposed or championed low impact licensing laws.

These seminal licensing laws would portend a problem that would haunt nursing in years to come. The new licensing laws essentially created different categories of nurses, all legal. There was the nurse who had a license and used the initials RN following her name. There was the individual who took a correspondence course and presented herself as a nurse. There was the individual who gained experience by caring for family and friends and was referred to as a nurse. The early licensing laws simply muddied the playing field. In 1914 Clara D. Noyes, then President of the National League of Nursing Education, addressed the issue of confusion caused by the licensing laws and the potential created for outside interference by special interests.

> For two years, a Committee for the American Hospital Association has been working upon a plan for grading nurses. As far as can be determined, it is an effort to classify the enormous body of women calling themselves nurses, trained and otherwise, and put them into different groups.(24)

The American Hospital Association did not succeed in their grading endeavor. The confusion continued until mid-century when mandatory licensing laws specifically identified who could legally practice as a nurse. However, by this time the question evolved from "who is a nurse" to "who is the professional nurse." Starting in the 1960s, the nursing establishment attempted to legislate who could legally practice as a "professional" nurse.

The nursing establishment in the United States never quite caught on to the spirit of the times. The spirit of reform was all around them, yet they seemed not to notice. They seemed *vacuumesque*. To the nursing elite, reform in nursing meant attaining professional status. To the practicing nurse, the toiler, reform in nursing meant bread, butter, and fewer hours of work. It is astounding such a large segment of American working women—toiler nurses—bypassed the Progressive Era without demanding reform. While they toiled away in their twelve-hour shifts and six and one-half day workweek, their leadership was on a crusade for professional status, not reform of working conditions. The leadership essentially betrayed their constituents. Gradually toiler nurses developed a subtle distrust of the nursing establishment. Eventually toiler nurses took matters into their own hands.

References

1. Gould, Louis L., editor. *The Progressive Era.* New York: Syracuse University Press. 1974. pg. 1
2. May, Ernest R. and the editors of *Life. The Progressive Era.* Volume 9. 1901–1917. Published by Time Incorporated. 1964. pg. 58.
3. *ibid.* pg. 59.
4. Schneider, Dorothy and Carl J. *American Women in the Progressive Era. 1900–1920.* New York: Anchor Books, Doubleday. 1993. pg. 4.
5. *ibid.* pg. 165.

6. Adickes, Sandra L. *To Be Young Was Very Heaven*. New York: St. Martins Press. 1997. pg. 88–90.

7. *ibid*. pgs. 5–6.

8. Orlick, Annelise. *Common Sense and a Little Fire*. Chapel Hill: University of North Carolina Press. 1995. pg. 53–54.

9. Schneider and Schneider. pg. 61–62.

10. Melosh, Barbara. *The Physicians Hand: Work, Culture and Conflict in American Nursing*. Philadelphia: Temple University Press. 1982. pg. 113.

11. Buhler-Wilkerson, Karen. "False Dawn: The Rise and Decline of Public Health Nursing in America, 1900–1930" in *Nursing History: New Perspectives, New Possibilities*. Ellen C. Lagemann, editor. New York: Teachers College Press. 1983. pg. 90.

12. Reverby, Susan. "Something Besides Waiting: The Politics of Private Duty Nursing Reform in the Depression" in *Nursing History: New Perspectives, New Possibilities*. Ellen C. Langemann, editor. New York: Teachers College Press. 1983. pg. 136.

13. Ashley, JoAnn. "Nursing and Early Feminism." *American Journal of Nursing*. September, 1975. pg. 1465.

14. "Some Urgent Social Claims" in *A Lavinia Dock Reader*. Janet Wilson James, editor. New York: Garland Publishing, Inc. 1985. pg. 899.

15. Lewenson, Sandra Beth. *Taking Charge: Nursing, Suffrage and Feminism in America, 1873–1920*. New York: Garland Publishing. 1993. pg. 175.

16. "Status of Women in the Working World" in *A Lavinia Dock Reader*. pgs. 971–975.

17. Melosh. pg. 98–99.

18. Reverby, Susan M. *Ordered to Care*. Cambridge, U.K.: Cambridge University Press. 1987. pg. 131.

19. Tomes, Nancy. "The Silent Battle: Nurse Registration in New York State, 1903-1920" in *Nursing History: New Perspectives, New Possibilities*. Ellen C. Langemann, editor. New York: Teachers College Press. 1983. pg. 110.

20. Schneider and Schneider. pgs. 14–16.

21. Tomes. pg. 117.

22. Kalish, Philip A. and Beatrice J. Kalish. *The Advance of American Nursing*. Philadelphia: J.B. Lippincott company. 3rd edition, 1995. pg. 193.

23. Tomes. pg. 109.

24. *Legacy of Leadership: Presidential Addresses from the Superintendents Society and NLNE, 1894–1952*. Nettie Birnbach and Sandra Lewenson, editors. New York: National League of Nursing Press. 1993. Publication # 14-2514. pg. 117.

6

STANDARDS FIRST, COUNTRY SECOND

The *Random House Webster's Dictionary* defines the word mystique in the following manner:

1. a framework of doctrines, beliefs, etc. constructed around a person or object and lending enhanced value or meaning.

2. an aura of mystery or mystical power surrounding a particular occupation or pursuit.

American nursing leaders of the twentieth century, particularly the academic types, really had mystique. Their accomplishments remain questionable, yet they sustained the interest and admiration of nurse historians. They failed to have nursing accepted as a profession, yet they succeeded in keeping the issue viable for an entire century. They were an elitist minority. They were unable to unify their goals with the bread and butter issues of the majority, the toiler nurse. However, they dominated the American nursing scene for the better part of the twentieth century. They convinced the nursing world the baccalaureate degree would bring professional recognition. Yet, while espousing the necessity of the latter, they introduced a two-year associate degree program.

Nursing history demonstrates one sure thing. There were inconsistencies in the behavior of the nursing leadership that bordered on the irrational. However, influential people listened when they spoke. WWI is a case in point. WWI, the nurse's aide problem, the American Red Cross, Adelaide Nutting, Annie Goodrich, and Jane Delano all intermingle in *the* grandstanding episode in the history of American nursing. The issues and the people came together and demonstrated the mystique of two well-known nursing educators. They were Adelaide Nutting and Annie Goodrich. These two women emerged from the Progressive Era relatively unscathed by anything *progressive*. However, during WWI they managed an inordinate degree of control over the supply of nursing personnel for the military.

But first, something about the times and context in which these women functioned. In WWI, unlike the situation in the Civil War, there was a semblance of an organized entity known as American nursing. In fact, this entity was referred to by some as the profession of nursing. Licensing laws, although permissive in nature, gave some nurses legal standing. There was some movement toward placement of nursing programs into collegiate settings. In 1909, the University of Minnesota established the first collegiate program for nurses. Unlike the Civil War Era when female physicians and genteel ladies were the leaders of nurses and nursing, there was now a nursing establishment. In contemporary parlance one could say, "You've come a long way, baby." Interestingly, many issues of contemporary nursing are issues that emerged in the timeframe of WWI. One such issue was the nurse's aide problem. To many, particularly members of the nursing establishment, nurse's aides did not have a place in nursing. Their presence was simply incompatible with the concept of nursing as a profession. Also, from a pecuniary perspective, nurse's aides represented competition. The permissive licensing laws allowed nurse's aides access to the type of patient considered the domain of the private duty nurse. This was the context when war was declared on Germany in April 1917.

With the declaration of war, Nutting immediately emerged from the academic setting at Teachers College, Columbia University, to assume leadership of the National Emergency Committee on Nursing. Nutting was concerned about rumors circulating to the effect that nursing school admission standards, graduation standards, and licensing requirements would be reduced in order to increase the supply of nurses available to meet civilian and military needs.(1) Always the educator and watchdog of the educational standards issue, Nutting was equally concerned about rumors from the European scene. There were stories of well to do young women taking short basic courses in nursing and rendering care in military hospitals. The romanticizing of war phenomenon was taking place among young women, and they wanted to serve in the military. In most cases their intent was only for the duration. However, it was reported that some of these women, once they returned to civilian life, demanded legal recognition as nurses. There was speculation the same scenario could occur in the United States. The ladies of the National Emergency Committee on Nursing perceived these rumors and speculation as real threats to prevailing nursing standards. This was their frame of mind as they assumed a role in meeting the civilian and military nursing needs of a nation at war.

The federal government was focusing on the supply and demand of nurses for the civilian home front and for the military at home and in Europe. The demand for nurses was great, and the responsibility to meet demands in both the civilian and military sectors was directed primarily to the American Red Cross. This organization served as the reserve for the Army and Navy Nurse Corps, established in 1901 and 1908 respectively. Jane Delano was head of the Red Cross Department of Nursing. Recruitment of nurses for the reserve was one of her major responsibilities. It was in this capacity that Delano clashed with the two academics—Nutting and Goodrich.

As this story unfolds, one should keep in mind the background of these individuals. Nutting and Goodrich were primarily educators. The specifics of Nutting's background were discussed in an earlier chapter. The majority of her career was spent as an educator in the confines of the prestigious Columbia University. Nutting was far removed from the day-to-day activities of the toiler nurse and did not have any direct accountability in meeting supply and demand issues associated with the war effort.

Annie Goodrich (1866–1954) had a somewhat more varied background. She had been a director of several hospital schools of nursing, worked with Lillian Wald of public health nursing fame, worked with Nutting at Columbia, and had been an inspector of nurse training schools in New York. She would become known in nursing circles as the dean of nursing because she became Dean of the Army School of Nursing and later the Yale University School of Nursing. Jane Delano (1862–1919) also had a varied background. She was a graduate of the Bellevue Hospital Training School for Nurses. She was an assistant superintendent of nurses at the University of Pennsylvania Hospital School of Nursing; she served as a superintendent of nurses at an emergency installation in Florida during the yellow fever epidemic and served as president of the Nurses' Associated Alumnae (later known as the ANA). She is recognized primarily for her work with the American Red Cross. Her most challenging responsibilities consisted of supplying nurses for the military during WWI and meeting the staffing demands of nursing services at the home front during the war and influenza epidemic of 1918–19.

The war duties of Nutting and Goodrich were advisory in nature. Delano had overall operational responsibility for the recruitment and deployment of nurses to appropriate assignments. Delano has been described as a practical idealist.(2) This description may also describe the motivating factor underlying Delano's approach to meeting the military's needs for nursing personnel.

In every war, there is the need to care for the soldier and for those he leaves behind in the civilian population. There is the battlefront and the homefront. Thus, the nursing needs increase substantially. The Army originally submitted a request to the Red Cross for 10,000 nurses. The request eventually reached a total of 35,000 nurses. (3) The wartime needs for additional nurses obviously had to be met from the civilian population. This in turn would deplete the number of nurses available to serve that population. Delano, the pragmatist, and Dora Thompson, superintendent of the Army Nurse Corps, advocated the utilization of nurse's aides in the military.(4) Initially the Surgeon General rejected the idea but reconsidered when needs became critical. He agreed to the utilization of nurse's aides in military facilities in the U.S.

The individuals would complete a four-week Red Cross basic nursing course and receive some additional practical training. They would be assigned only to the convalescent patient.(5) This was a reasonable plan. Nutting and Goodrich became aware of the plan, and all hell broke loose. The issue as perceived by Nutting and Goodrich was simply a matter of standards. It was their point of view only those individuals who graduated from a state-approved program and were licensed by the state (RN) should be eligible for military service. It has been recorded that Nutting said that inexperienced nurses should not care for wounded and dying men, and she borrowed President's Wilson's comment that war was not for amateurs.(6)

There were also other concerns regarding the nurse's aide proposal. If women completed the Red Cross course for aides, they would be ready for assignment in a matter of weeks. Nutting and Goodrich feared that young women who might ordinarily become students in a three-year nursing program would opt for the much shorter Red

Cross Course. Also, the nurse's aide would receive $30 a month. The short course and the stipend were an attractive opportunity for many young women.

In view of the existing permissive licensing laws, the ladies of the nursing establishment also feared the impact trained nurses' aides would have on the post-war environment. Delano, Nutting, and Goodrich presented their positions and concerns at a joint meeting of nursing organizations in May 1918. The organizations represented were the National League of Nursing Education, the American Nurses Association, and the National Organization for Public Health Nursing.

There was an added dimension to what was now being labeled a controversy.(7) Goodrich was proposing an Army School of Nursing in lieu of the nurses' aide program proposed by Delano. This would be a dream come true for the ladies of the nursing establishment. The proposal called for a three-year diploma program aligned with the Office of the Surgeon General and under the supervision of a dean who would have overall administrative responsibility. The school would be independent of any hospital administrator. The training units would be hospital facilities at individual campsites. The curriculum would meet requirements for state registration and each training area would have its own faculty. Upon completion of the three-year program the graduate would go into the Army Nurse Corps. The principal advocates of this plan never explained how this three-year yet to be initiated program would satisfy the immediate nursing needs of the military.

Delano had her opportunity at this meeting and expressed the following:

I cannot believe that we should use at this time the services of our graduate nurses to sit down and feed helpless men in the war; I believe that woman of common sense or judgment ... could do these services acceptably, and that a very grave responsibility will rest upon us if ultimately we prevent from drawing into the hospitals a number of women, trained students or aides to meet the military needs.(8)

This was Delano the pragmatist and the person responsible for providing personnel to meet the nursing needs of the military. Keep in mind Delano's proposal called for the nurses' aides to provide care for convalescent patients, not the acutely ill or injured. Physicians attended this joint meeting of nursing organizations and made their comments for and against the Goodrich proposal. Dr. Winford Smith, a colonel in the Surgeon General's Office, spoke on behalf of the Army School of Nursing. His comments reflect concern for obtaining the "right type of woman" for the nursing ranks. In reference to a higher level of entrance requirements usually not seen in the civilian schools, he said the following:

It will likewise guarantee to us a type mentally and morally best fitted to our service.(9)

The Delano camp had their physician spokesman in the person of S.S. Goldwater, M.D. He was director, Mount Sinai Hospital; Service Committee, American Hospital Association; chairman, Committee on Hospitals, General Medical Board, Council of National Defense. Dr. Goldwater was deeply concerned. He viewed the nursing situation as a crisis not only for the military but also for the civilian hospitals. He feared that the proposed Army School of Nursing would attract students who would ordinarily go into the civilian hospital schools, thus depleting the number of nurses caring for the civilian population. He said the following:

> The truth of the matter is that the country cannot spare the number of graduate nurses that the Army requires, nor can the training schools produce new graduates in sufficient numbers to satisfy the needs of both the military and the civil population.(10)

Goldwater went on in a practical tone and reminded the group that Surgeon General Gorgas was not in favor of the Army School proposal.

> If the large numbers that are expected to enroll were not an *additional* supply, but were merely drawn away from the civil hospitals, the civil hospitals and the civilian population would suffer immediately. On the other hand, if the number of enrollments were small, the whole project would fail to satisfy the Army's pressing needs. These were undoubtedly some of the reasons that led Surgeon General Gorgas to declare, in an official memorandum dated January 24th, 1918, that "the plan of organizing training schools in connection with Army hospitals is not believed to be practical."(11)

Goldwater not only supported the nurse's aide program, he knew exactly the type of individual he wanted in the program.

The women that I have in mind belong wholly or almost wholly to the leisure class. They are now contributing nothing to the efficiency of the nation or to the success of the war; yet they are strong healthy, patriotic, and willing. They are the only labor reserve that the country possesses, and they can be brought into the nursing field without lessening the supply of workers for any essential industry. They want to serve the nation, and they should be permitted to do so. The same class is giving valuable service in England; England would be lost, and we shall be lost, without them. When the war is over, the nursing aides will melt away into private life, strengthened and chastened by their experience, leaving the nursing field in the hands of professional nurses. They should be prepared now, for in no other way can the war nursing problem is solved.(12)

Goldwater was addressing an audience in 1918 and his perception of women of the leisure class was probably accurate. They were an available resource who could provide basic nursing care for a nation desperate for such services. The skills they needed could be attained in an acceptable period of time—four weeks. It was a reasonable plan of action. However, the mystique of Nutting and Goodrich was alive and well. The conventioneers supported the Army School of Nursing.

The Army School of Nursing proposal was rejected by the War Department. The nursing establishment in the persons of Nutting and Goodwrich sought the intervention of the Secretary of War, and he overturned the decision of the War Department. The proposal received approval on May 25, 1918. Annie Goodrich was appointed Dean. The first recruitment literature was issued June 7, 1918 and the Armistice was signed November 11, 1918. The commencements for the first graduating classes of the Army School of Nursing were in June and July of 1921. Mary Roberts, in her comprehensive history text titled *American Nursing* points out by 1923 the School had been reduced to one site, the Walter Reed General Hospital.(13) The School closed in August 1931. Roberts indicates the reasons were economic conditions, high cost of nursing affiliations and the lack of acceptance by the Army Nurse Corps.(14) A total of 937 women completed the course of study at the Army School of Nursing. Five hundred of these women were in the first graduating class of 1921. (15) The remaining 437 graduated in the 1921–1931 timeframe. These were not impressive numbers. Roberts states Goodrich acknowledged the number of students did not make an appreciable contribution to the war effort and presents a quote by Goodrich that is simply disingenuous. Goodrich, speaking of what she now viewed as the "experiment," is quoted as follows:

> ...it demonstrated without doubt the great asset a well established school under the Medical Department would be in the rapid expansion of nursing service required by a similar emergency.(16)

The statement is completely inaccurate as indicated by the numbers alone. It was probably a rationalization by Goodrich to accommodate for the obvious failure of her project. With the advent of WWII, there was once again an increased demand for nurses. However, there was no support for rekindling the Army School.(17) This was a significant blow to Goodrich. Harriet Koch, in *The Militant Angel,* writes that Goodrich was extremely disappointed when, in WWII, the Council of Nursing Education disavowed the Army School of Nursing and instituted the United States Cadet Nurse Corps.(18) This latter and successful enterprise was the antithesis of the Army School of Nursing and will be discussed in a subsequent chapter.

The nursing history texts describe yet another educational program supposedly aimed at meeting the nation's nursing requirements during WWI. This endeavor involved Vassar College, a women's college in Poughkeepsie, New York. In reality it had more to do with the private agenda of the nursing establishment. Specifically, the underlying issue of this program was about status. The endeavor was the Vassar Training Camp for Nurses, sometimes referred to as Vassar's Rainbow Division. The original idea is credited to a Mrs. John Blodgett, a Vassar trustee. Her concept was to train college women as nurses' aides. She apparently sought advice from Nutting and soon had a change of concept.(19) Nutting, the academic, saw the Vassar Training Camp as a way of connecting college women and nursing. This would meet Nutting's idea of the right type of woman, thus elevating the status of nursing.

The Vassar Training Camp provided a three-month preparatory course at the Vassar Campus. The student would then complete the nursing program at a participating hospital. The students wore the uniform of their particular hospital; thus the different colors of the uniforms led to the designation of Rainbow Division. Because advance credit was given for their college work, the student could complete the program in two years and three months. Like the Army School of Nursing, there would not be any immediate benefit to the nation. Like the Army School of Nursing, the Vassar project cannot be considered a success. Less than half of the 431 students finished the program.(20) Many left the program with the signing of the Armistice, which occurred only months following the initiation of the camp. Nutting had pursued the romantic college girl who wanted to serve for the duration only.

What can be said in summation regarding World War I and nursing leadership in America? It should be obvious even to the casual reader of nursing history that the quest for professional status was their overriding concern. This concern overshadowed the needs of a nation at war, a nation desperate for additional nurse power. The Army School of Nursing provided the coveted autonomy that came with freedom from hospital administrators. The Vassar Program provided the coveted affiliation with a college and college-educated women. Both programs provided greater access to women who met enhanced admission criteria, so important to the status issue. Essentially, Nutting and Goodrich utilized the war as a means to the status end.

The question remains how these women were able to exert such influence? Was it, as described by Goldwater, a matter of their zeal, perseverance, determination, one-sided intensity, and mild hysterics?(21) Did the Secretary of War perceive these women as Florence Nightingale incarnates? Did he recall the history of the Crimean War? Did he remember the public insult the military establishment endured as a result of Nightingale's revelations regarding the poor standard of care for the British soldier? Did he perceive these women as having the moral high ground and heaven help those who did not do their bidding? Perhaps the American military establishment realized the war was reaching a conclusion, and it was simply pragmatic to let the ladies have their own way. All these factors probably contributed to the mystique of the nursing leaders, allowing them undue influence in crucial matters affecting a nation at war.

A few more insights concerning "the nurses' aide problem." The state of the art of nursing during the World War I timeframe was such that utilization of nurses' aides made perfect sense. Unlike today, high technology in the delivery of nursing care was not an issue. In most instances nursing care consisted of meeting the basic needs of the human being, i.e., feeding, bathing, providing assistance with elimination needs, and providing a safe and secure environment. The procedures used by the nurse in patient care were not complex in nature. The properly trained nurses' aide could handle most of the nursing procedures of the day. The nurse could best be used in a supervisory capacity and assisting with or performing more complex procedures such as an extensive wound dressing.

The nursing establishment ignored these facts. Most likely they were still held hostage to the Sairy Gamp image of nurses. These leaders were not far removed from the Nightingale era, during which the quality of nurses and nursing care was definitely lacking. However, by 1918 the care of the sick and those rendering care had improved substantially and were subjected to increased public scrutiny. In their campaign against Delano's nurse's aide proposal, the ladies of the nursing establishment expressed concern about potential post-war problems. Nurses' aides would supposedly flood the nursing market and claim their Red Cross training afforded them the title of nurse.

Perhaps more anxiety-provoking to the nursing establishment was the potential phenomena addressed by Dorothy Johnson in her book titled *History and Trends of Practical Nursing*. She describes two concerns that could account for nurses' aide bashing. Given small tasks initially, the nurse's aide could gradually assume more responsibility and eventually usurp the position of the nurse. Another possible concern was the length of the training programs of both nurses and nurse's aides. The three-year hospital training program could be in jeopardy if a nurse's aide, while spending less time in formal learning, successfully perform basic nursing care.(22)

However, the bogus issue of this saga was Nutting's concern about European women serving as nurses' aides in military hospitals in Europe. Who were these women Nutting feared could ruin American Nursing? They were known officially as VADs—Voluntary Aide Detachments. They were the romantic types; they were usually well-to-do young European women who had no intention of subjecting themselves to the rigors of training associated with the toiler nurse. It is difficult to believe, as did Nutting, that post-war these women would return to their homes and demand legal recognition to function as nurses in such countries as status conscious Great Britain. These were women of the leisure class, the types Goldwater pleaded for in his address supporting Delano's aide proposal. These women would not be returning to civilian life as your average working girl.

Julia C. Stimson, RN, was an American Army Chief Nurse in a British hospital in France. She held a demanding and responsible position. Following the war she published a book titled *Finding Themselves*.(23) In the book, a compilation of letters describing the daily routine of the unit, she expresses her feelings regarding the utilization of nurses' aides. She said, in part, the following:

> ...word has been sent back to the United States that we need more help. I should like sixty-five more Red Cross nurses from St. Louis, or if I can't have them, sixty-five of the nurse's aides that we trained. They would certainly find here a sufficient outlet for their energies. They could be of the greatest help, and on the whole I do not know but that I should rather have the aides that I know than a lot of trained nurses that I do not know. (24)

Stimson was echoing the state of affairs that Delano was trying to resolve. Help was needed at the bedside, and the person of the nurse's aide could easily provide such help. This additional "need for help" theme would echo throughout twentieth century nursing, and the same type of response from the nursing establishment would be forthcoming—train more professional nurses.

Delano experienced many insults from Nutting and Goodrich regarding the nurse's aide issue. In many aspects she resembles Linda Richards. Like Richards, she was criticized for being too practical. Like Richards, she held very important administrative positions. Delano provided a vital service for a country at war in her position with the Red Cross. She did not have the worries of an academic nurse such as Nutting or Goodrich. She had concerns of a more practical nature. She had to provide the doers, the people to actually render the nursing care to patients. Kernodle described her in the following manner.

> Miss Delano was a practical idealist; she liked people, and she wished to do good. She had a nature both broad and deep but not complex, with ambitions that were clear-cut and simple. Since she was not a devotee of causes like Lavinia Dock, a thinker and educator like Miss Nutting or Miss Goodrich, or a woman absorbed in the complex interests of her profession like Clara D. Noyes, it is likely that the more intellectual wing of the profession did not find her entirely congenial; but on a personal level almost anyone would respond to the warmth, genuineness and strength of her personality.(25)

This simple, not complex woman is buried in Arlington National Cemetery.

References

1. Donahue, Patricia M. *Nursing the Finest Art.* St. Louis: C.V. Mosby Company. 1985. pg. 398.
2. Kernodle, Portia B. *The Red Cross Nurse in Action—1882–1948.* New York: Harper & Brothers, 1949. pg. 49.

3. Kalish, Philip A. and Beatrice J. Kalish. *The Advance of American Nursing.* Philadelphia: J.B. Lippincott Company. 3rd edition, 1995. pg. 216.

4. *ibid.* pg. 224.

5. *ibid.*

6. *ibid.*

7. Koch. Harriet B. *Militant Angel.* New York: Macmillan Company. 1951. pg. 93.

9. As quoted in Kalish and Kalish. pg. 226.

10. Goldwater. S.S. "The Nursing Crisis: Efforts to Satisfy the Nursing Requirements of the War. A Way out of the Difficulty." Comments presented at the Twenty-First Annual Convention. *American Journal of Nursing.* Volume 18. (1918) pg. 1030-1036.

11. *ibid.* pg. 1035.

12. *ibid.* pg. 1036.

13. Roberts, Mary M. *American Nursing.* New York: The Macmillan Company. 1954. pg. 140.

14. *ibid.*

15. Donahue. pg. 402.

16. Roberts, pg. 140.

17. *ibid.*

18. Koch. pg. 141.

19. Stewart, Isabel M. "Nursing Preparedness" *American Journal of Nursing* Volume 41. (July, 1941). pg. 812.

20. Clappison, Gladys B. *Vassar's Rainbow Division, 1918.* Iowa: The Graphic Publishing Company, Inc. 1964. pgs. 135; 352–353.

21. Kernodle. pg. 139.

22. Johnson, Dorothy F. *History and Trends of Practical Nursing.* St. Louis: C.V. Mosby. 1966. pg. 43.

23. Stimson, Julia C. *Finding Themselves.* New York: The Macmillan Company, 1918.

24. *ibid.* pg. 34.

25. Kernodle, pg. 49.

7

SOME DEFINING MOMENTS

The decades of the 1920s and 1930s were difficult times for all Americans. There was the Great Depression. Because of this event, the person known as the hospital staff nurse emerged. During this timeframe, nurses demonstrated an interest in the labor movement. American society demonstrated an awareness that something was amiss in the field of nursing and initiated a series of commissions to determine and correct that something. America and nursing once again prepared for war. These events would define American nursing for the remainder of the twentieth century. Times were changing and the nursing establishment was getting nervous. They sensed a lack of influence and control in shaping the destiny of American nursing.

The Great Depression sent nursing into a tailspin. The era of the private duty nurse passed. She was a luxury no one could afford. Many, many nurses were without employment, and they were desperate. They offered their services to hospitals and accepted room and board as payment for services rendered; thus, the entry of the hospital staff nurse onto the hospital scene. Many hospital schools of nursing closed. Hospital administrators discovered it was cheaper to close schools and utilize the services of the employment starved staff nurse. The Great Depression passed and the economic conditions of the hospital industry improved. However the working conditions of the hospital nurse remained the same. She was still working the Depression Era schedule of twelve-hour shifts and a six and one-half day week. She began to complain about working conditions. It was the 1930s, and it was the beginning of union activity among the ranks Dock called the toiler nurse. The American Federation of Labor (AFL) and the Congress of Industrial Organizations (CIO) began recruitment of nurses.(1) In New York City, the Hospital and Medical Employees, CIO, organized the municipal hospital nurses and negotiated an eight-hour day. (2) This was significant. The labor movement had arrived on the nursing scene. Following WWII the labor movement would become an integral part of American nursing. It would not cause but would contribute to the internal chaos that plagued American nursing for the remainder of the century.

When all else fails appoint a commission, conduct a study, and issue a report. That is the American way. In the early twentieth century, the medical establishment followed this design and produced the Flexner Report. This report garnered public opinion in favor of reform and produced a substantial increase of foundation monies into medical education.(3) These results were exactly what the nursing establishment perceived as essential for the advancement of nursing education. Also, they psychologically identified with many of the specific recommendations of the Flexner Report, particularly the following:

1. There has been an over-production of poorly trained medical practitioners.

2. The existence of large numbers of commercial medical schools was the primary cause of the over-production of poorly trained medical practitioners.

3. There needed to be fewer yet better equipped and better operated medical schools.

4. The medical school should articulate with the university and general system of education.(4)

These recommendations reflected parallel concerns of the nursing establishment regarding nursing education. There were too many hospitals with inferior schools of nursing, which were producing poorly prepared nurses who were flooding the labor market. This created a negative impact on the image of nursing, resulting in recruitment problems for the higher-caliber schools. The nursing establishment desperately wanted the teaching of nursing out of the hospital and into the college setting.

The Flexner Report was published in 1910. In 1911, Nutting approached the Carnegie Foundation for funding for a similar study of nursing, but was essentially ignored. (5)

It was 1919 before Nutting convinced the Rockefeller Foundation to fund the study that would be known as the Goldmark Report. It was anticipated the Goldmark Report would do for nursing education what the Flexner Report supposedly did for medical education. The report would identify problems within nursing, the individuals responsible for the problems, and remedies that would correct the problems. However, the scenario never played out in this fashion. Throughout the twentieth century many official reports with specific recommendations were issued in response to issues plaguing nursing and nursing education. However, many significant and important recommendations were never acted upon by the nursing establishment. The nursing establishment simply did not agree with many of the recommendations, and inaction was their preferred response. However, the nursing establishment agreed with some recommendations, particularly those fostering the move of nursing education into the academic setting. The fact was they lacked a forum and authority to initiate even those changes they viewed in a positive manner.

Nursing and Nursing Education in the United States, referred to as the Goldmark Report in deference to the principal investigator Josephine Goldmark, was published in 1922. The report reinforced what the nursing establishment had been saying for years. It concluded the majority of hospital training programs were not adequate for training purposes and the students' education was secondary to the needs of the hospital. It acknowledged the need for the school of nursing to be independent of hospital administration.

However, the authors of the report viewed the hospital training school as the proper site for teaching the nursing of acute diseases; the university school should prepare nurses for public health nursing, hospital supervision, and nursing education.(6) This last finding, the separation of nursing education into hospital and university settings is very important in the telling of the story of American nursing. The committee, in effect, was identifying two types of nursing education and two types of nursing practice. There would be technical education for technical practice in the hospital setting. There would be an academic education for those not involved in direct nursing care in the hospital setting. Similar recommendations would be made by subsequent commissions throughout the twentieth century. However, the nursing establishment never seriously considered implementation of these recommendations calling for a two-pronged approach to nursing education and practice.

Why the recalcitrance regarding recommendations of this nature? The nursing establishment would lose any semblance of control of hospital nursing education and nursing practice if they accepted the division of nursing into two formats. The nursing establishment would be relegated to the academic domain, controlling a small minority of nurses. The nursing establishment maintained ambivalent feelings toward the hospital or toiler nurse. Although the nursing establishment disliked the image of the toiler nurse, they loved their perception of controlling the largest segment of practicing nurses.

The Goldmark Report made additional recommendations contrary to the official viewpoint of the nursing leadership.

There appears to be a real place in nursing service of a subsidiary type, for the routine care of patients suffering from disease of a mild or chronic type or in convalescence.(7)

Once again the topic of nurses' aides was suggested as a method of meeting patients' basic nursing needs. Once again, like the fracas over the aide issue in WWI, the nursing establishment would not entertain such a proposal. They maintained a subsidiary worker of any kind would threaten nursing standards. History indicates the nursing establishment considered Goldmark too concerned with efficiency issues.(8)

The Goldmark Report did not have a significant impact on nursing. Historical speculation is the report lacked influence because all nursing schools were not surveyed. At the time of survey, there were over 1,800 nursing schools and Goldmark surveyed 23.(9) The Flexner Report, the prototype, was a survey of all 155 medical schools in the US and Canada. It is inconceivable Goldmark, even with the assistance of committee members, could have conducted the same type of study as Flexner. Sheer numbers worked against such an endeavor. The limited impact probably had more to do with the lack of any type of official body to direct implementation. The ladies of the nursing establishment lacked official standing, except among themselves.

In 1926, another attempt was made to conduct a study of nursing education in the United States. The National League of Nursing Education (NLNE) spearheaded this endeavor. The official title of this group was the Committee on the Grading of Nursing Schools. This study was to do what Goldmark failed to accomplish—the grading or classification of nursing schools. The anticipation was poor caliber hospital schools of nursing would receive low grades when compared to the more prestigious schools. Once the results of the study were published, the public would demand the closing of the inferior schools of nursing.

This was not exactly what happened. The committee took on a life of its own. What started as a five-year project lasted eight years. The committee expanded the study and added two additional goals. Besides the grading of schools, they would study the supply and demand issue and they would conduct a job analysis.(10) However, like Goldmark, they did not personally survey schools of nursing. Instead they relied on extensive questionnaires for their data.

For various reasons no attempt was made to grade or classify the schools. Roberts states the committee believed it would be unfair to some schools, regardless of the quality of the school.(11) Goldenberg reasons it is because they failed to conduct a specific school-by-school analysis.(12) Reverby quotes a variety of possibilities such as difficulty in obtaining accurate data without onsite visits; the arbitrary nature of classification programs; and lack of consensus on what constituted good standards.(13) These resemble rationalizations. The most probable reason was pressure exerted on the grading committee by the power groups of the day, specifically the American Medical Association (AMA) and the American Hospital Association (AHA). The AMA and AHA did not want closure of any schools of nursing because student nurses were still the major providers of nursing care to hospitalized patients. If a grading report was published the public would demand the closure of identified inferior schools cited in the report. Helen E. Marshall, in her biography of Nutting, quotes the nurse leader as saying the following about the committee.

> The results of the study are of little consequence, the cost of the seven years labor has been enormous, and the expense of the meetings has been little short of a disgrace, to those in charge of a responsible piece of professional investigation and reform.(14)

Thus history records another expensive impotent study of American nursing. However, the Committee on the Grading of Schools of Nursing published a total of three reports that demonstrated some basic insights regarding problems within nursing. One of those reports, *Nurses, Patients and Pocketbooks*, made some pertinent observations.

> Hospitals run training schools for two reasons. the first reason is that it is cheaper to run a poor school than it is to employ graduate nurses. ... The second reason why hospitals conduct training schools and this probably applies to most of the large and famous schools, as well as to many small ones, is that it is easier

to handle the nursing service of a hospital with student nurses than with graduate nurses.(15)

Statements such as these validated what the nursing establishment knew to be the reality for nurses in the hospital situation. And in 1918 Nutting stated that Henry James would consider hospital-training programs the "moral equivalent of war."(16).

Statements such as these failed to challenge the nursing establishment into action. They maintained their passive-aggressive behavior and continued to bemoan the situation. After the publication of several major reports, there was still no effort to actively challenge the ills of apprenticeship nurse training and the working conditions of the emerging staff nurse. These reports were a product of the 1920s, the immediate decade following the Progressive Era.

Didn't anything rub off on these leaders? At some point the ladies of the establishment should have said "enough" and turned to the labor movement for support. They failed to do this because of the professional issue. Also, the nursing establishment of the day was comprised mainly of educators who were probably not comfortable with nuts and bolts issues associated with everyday nursing in the hospital situation.

In 1910, Robb died tragically in a street car accident. This left Nutting as the titular head of American nursing. Her world was the world of academe not the world of the toiler nurse. Like many educators, her perspective on rectifying the major problems of nursing was monetary in nature. She said, "The root of all the main problems in nursing will be found, I believe, if carefully studied to be economic in nature."(17) In 1916 she told the New York State Nurses Association the following:

> I firmly believe that generous financial help would flow into our training schools from private sources were the need fully recognized, and I see no reason whatever why schools rendering an important public service should not also secure substantial aid from public funds."(18)

Nutting was quite familiar with the Flexner Report and the consequent infusion of monies into American medical education. She probably hoped American nursing would have similar good fortune. Her reference regarding the use of public funds is interesting. Did she secretly entertain the idea that the education of nurses should come under the public domain? Nutting knew the nursing situation was not improving. She was simply unable to get down and dirty and start agitating for solutions.

The major reports previously mentioned and many reports of the future would support utilization of a subsidiary worker in nursing. As discussed earlier, the standards issue and fear of competition motivated both the nursing establishment and toiler nurses to maintain opposition to subsidiary workers. In fact, it was probably one of the few issues about which the two groups agreed. The reality was such a worker had always been part of the nursing scene and assumed increased significance during the modern era of American nursing. They were identified by various titles, the most common being nurse's aide, nursing attendant, and practical nurse. They usually found employment in the home, caring for the sick, cleaning the patient's environment, and making meals. For the most part subsidiary workers received on-the-job training, although some took advantage of short courses sponsored by hospitals or the American Red Cross. These caregivers were unlicensed nursing personnel. Statistical data is not available regarding the numbers and types of employment in which these persons engaged during the timeframe immediately preceding WWII. However, one author estimates, in 1940, there were 190,000 such individuals engaged in the field of nursing.(19)

The term "practical nurse" did not always have formal meaning as it does today. It originally applied to individuals who performed basic nursing care. However, the state of New York changed that in 1938, when a new licensing law was enacted. The new law required mandatory licensing of practical nurses and established regulations concerning practical schools of nursing. The licensed practical nurse (LPN) was now on her way to a permanent and important presence in American nursing and the hospital industry.

In 1941, she was also becoming a thorn in the side of the RN. WWII, like all other wars, caused a serious nursing shortage at the home front, and the LPN filled many of the vacancies ordinarily filled by RNs. Also, the War Nursing Council, a wartime coalition of nursing organizations, endorsed the training of practical nurses. Unlike the WWI era, individuals such as Nutting and Goodrich did not emerge to cast aspersion on these caregivers. In fact nursing leaders of the WWII generation were relatively silent on the issue of subsidiary workers of any category.

No one lobbied government officials for their official demise as members of the nursing team.

The lack of an antagonist to subsidiary workers was recognition their services were critical for the home front. It was also recognition that many of the nursing skills held sacrosanct by RNs could be accomplished by individuals with less training. During WWII the American Red Cross and the Office of Civilian Defense trained more than 200,000 volunteer nurses' aides.(20) As in the Crimean and American Civil Wars, the military experience of WWII had a lasting effect.

In fact, the military experience in WWII extended to American nursing a model for the delivery of nursing care in the civilian sector. The military utilized the RN in a very effective manner. The RN was the acknowledged leader of the nursing team. She taught and supervised the enlisted personnel who administer the direct nursing care. This method proved efficient and effective. However, in the post war years the nursing establishment would not accept this system. They still refused to accept subsidiary workers as legitimate team members. The practical nurse and to a greater extent the nurse's aide/nursing attendant continued to struggle for acceptance as contributing members of the nursing team. Dependent upon the recurring cycles of nursing shortages, both groups would experience peaks and valleys in hospital employment. However, both groups had demonstrated their effectiveness when utilized in the appropriate assignment.

WWI had the Army School of Nursing and the Vassar Training Camp. WWII had the U.S. Cadet Nurse Corps. All three endeavors were the vehicles by which a country at war attempted to meet the civilian and military demand for nurses. The WWI endeavors were driven by the personalities of Goodrich and Nutting. A congresswoman from Ohio, Frances Payne Bolton, drove the WWII endeavor. The WWI endeavors were failures, and the WWII endeavor was a success. The difference was plain old common sense and expediency. Goodrich and Nutting created new programs to meet the emergency. Bolton utilized a well-entrenched system—the hospital apprenticeship training program. The Nurse Training Act of 1943, also known as the Bolton Act, created the U.S. Cadet Nurse Corps. This was the first major federal subsidization of nursing education in America.

It was also a major and successful recruitment endeavor. The country needed nurses. The military had nearly drained the civilian nursing segment of its critical mass. The objective was to put as many student nurses as possible into hospital training programs. The student nurses, while receiving their training, would be replacing the civilian staff nurses who left for military service. The student was completely subsidized and received a monthly stipend. Her obligation was to serve in an appropriate civilian or military assignment for the duration of the war and six months. The program came under the auspices of the United States Public Health Service and the program director reported to the Surgeon General. "From its inception to its termination, The Cadet Nurse Corps had enrolled 169,443 student nurses in 1,125 of the nation's 1,300 nursing schools. Of these, 124,065 saw their training through to graduation."(21)

The attrition rate for the Cadet Program was significantly lower than the programs of the WWI era. Nurse historian Roberts discusses the attrition rate. She points out that the wartime class of the Army School of Nursing graduated less than one-third of the class. In contrast, the wartime classes of the Cadet Program graduated two-thirds of the enrolled students. Roberts struggles to rationalize this contrast. She tells us the Army School students were older, had well-developed occupational interests, and were in school only one year before conclusion of hostilities. She fails to analyze how these variables explain the attrition rate. She goes on to speculate that the students of the Army School were not favorably impressed with the military hospitals, whereas the cadet student nurse of WWII viewed her training hospital as part of the social structure of her community.(22)

Perhaps it comes down to less romanticism about WWII and lack of any major influence on the part of the nurse academics. Expectations for cadets were quite specific—the duration and six months. The leadership of the Cadet Nurse Corps was focused. "The Bolton Act is designed to increase the available nursepower of the country by preparing more nurses more rapidly."(23) So stated Lucile Petrie, RN, director of the U.S. Cadet Nurse Corps and later the first woman assistant surgeon general of the United States Public Health Service. The U.S. government spent a great deal of money on this project and demanded and got results.

The cult of professionalism consumed the nursing leadership since the beginning of the twentieth century. By the 1920s, it was evident adherence to this doctrine was stifling the progress of nursing. Major reports were issued about conditions in nursing and nursing education. It was now publicly acknowledged that student nurses were essentially laborers in a hospital system. Goldmark recommended a subsidiary worker. This so incensed the nursing leadership that they attacked Goldmark as being soft on standards. Another group, the Committee on the Grading of Schools of Nursing issued three reports but not *the* one report that would have a major impact on nursing, a grading report. Still, the leadership did nothing.

Nutting went the verbal complaint route, but failed to take any definitive action and essentially retired from the active nursing scene. The failure of the reports to initiate changes in nursing was undoubtedly a great disappointment to Nutting. Her naiveté and a little grandiosity caused her to believe there could be a Flexner Report for nursing. Such a report, upon publication, would expose the ills and evils of apprenticeship nurse training, and legions of reformers would come forward and save the day. A report, saying just the right thing, could put nursing on the road to recognition as a profession. After all, that's what the Flexner Report did for medical education.

The reality was that there was little shared between medical and nursing education. Failure to recognize this stymied the progress of nursing in terms of unity of purpose and general advancement. Not accepting subsidiary workers added to the remoteness of the nursing establishment. In WWII, the Red Cross and the federal government took matters into their own hands and trained sufficient numbers of subsidiary workers for the war emergency. The practical nurse and nurse's aide made inroads as members of the nursing team. During WWII, the military successfully employed the nursing team model. All this was accomplished without official support from the nursing establishment. Their belief system regarding standards and professional status was a serious hindrance to the progress of American nursing. This became increasingly evident as time progressed. Also, certain segments within American nursing were defining themselves, and the nursing establishment had nothing to say about it.

The ultimate sacrifice made by the nursing establishment in the name of professionalism was the failure to recognize the need for assistance from the labor movement. Wagner put it rather bluntly. "Hospital nursing, stripped of its prestige from close association with doctors and medical technology, bears similarities to factory work. The contradiction between this reality and professional nursing's rhetoric is as constant a battle today as it was in the 1932–1946 period."(24) This statement was made in 1980. During the second half of the twentieth century the toiler nurse increasingly sought assistance from unions. The nursing establishment increasingly sought solace within the academic setting.

References

1. Melosh, Barbara. *The Physicians Hand*. Philadelphia: Temple University Press. 1982. pg. 198.
2. Wagner, David. "The Proletarianization of Nursing in the U.S." *International Journal of Health Services*. Volume 10. #2. 1980. pg. 283.

3. Garling, Jean. "Flexner and Goldmark: Why the Difference in Impact"? *Nursing Outlook.* Volume 33. #1. (Jan-Feb) 1985. pg. 27.

4. Flexner, Abraham. *Medical Education in the United States and Canada.* A Report to the Carnegie Foundation for the Advancement of Teaching. New York: Arno Press and the New York Times. 1977. From the introduction by Henry S. Pritchett.

5. Kalish, Philip A. and Beatrice J. Kalish. *The Advance of American Nursing.* Philadelphia: J.B. Lippincott Company. 3rd edition. 1995. pg. 197.

6. Committee for the Study of Nursing Education. *Nursing and Nursing Education in the United States and a Report of a Survey* by Josephine Goldmark, Secretary. New York: The Macmillan Company, 1923. pg. 28.

7. *ibid.* pg. 26.

8. Goldenberg, Gary. *Nurses of a Different Stripe.* New York: Columbia University School of Nursing. 1992. pg. 106.

9. *ibid.*

10. Roberts, Mary M. *American Nursing.* New York: Macmillan Company, 1954. pg. 185.

11. *ibid.* pg. 186.

12. Goldenberg. pg. 108.

13. Reverby, Susan M. *Ordered to Care.* Cambridge, U.K.: Cambridge University Press. 1987. pg. 174.

14. Marshall, Helen F. *Mary Adelaide Nutting: Pioneer of Modern Nursing.* Baltimore: John Hopkins University Press. 1972. pg. 347.

15. Committee on the Grading of Nursing Schools. *Nurses, Patients and Pocketbooks.* A Report of a Study of the

Economics of Nursing. Mary Ayers Burgess, Director. New York: The Committee. 1928

16. Nutting, Mary Adelaide. *A Sound Economic Basis for Schools of Nursing and Other Addresses.* New York: Garland Publishing, Inc. 1984. pg. 354.

17. *ibid.* From the preface vi.

18. *ibid.* pg. 15.

19. Johnson, Dorothy F. *History and Trends of Practical Nursing.* Saint Louis: C.V. Mosby Company, 1966. pg. 40.

20. Bullough, Bonnie. "The Lasting Impact of World War 2 on Nursing." *American Journal of Nursing.* January, 1976. pg. 120.

21. United States Public Health Service. *The United States Cadet Nurse Corps (1943–1948) and other Federal Nurse Training Programs.* Washington, D.C. 1950. pg. 78.

22. Roberts. pg. 388.

23. Petry, Lucille. "The U.S. Cadet Nurse Corps—A Summing Up." *American Journal of Nursing.* December, 1945. pg. 1027.

24. Wagner. pg. 289.

8

MORE REPORTS, MORE RECALCITRANCE

The time frame is the twenty-five years following WWII. Still absent is an individual or organization that could legitimately claim they represented the collective body known as American nursing. The ANA was evolving into a labor organization. The NLN's only interest remained educational issues. The National Council of State Boards of Nursing was not yet a reality. Also absent were leaders with the persistence of Nutting or Goodrich or the firebrand of Dock. Nurses who earned name recognition were usually nurse educators. They were essentially personalities, espousing their personal viewpoints regarding theories of nursing, curriculum development, characteristics of a professional nurse, etc. The dichotomy between the academic and practice groups was now quite evident. Also quite evident was the major concern of the nursing establishment. It was the education of the nurse, not the nursing of patients.

The Great Depression and WWII brought a hiatus
in commissions and reports dealing with the trials and
tribulations of nurses and nursing. In 1948, society again
demonstrated a willingness to assist American nursing in
putting their house in order. Several new reports were
published and some were prescriptive in nature. Problems
were identified, and blueprints were established for
resolution. The reports dealt with education and some
practice issues.

Two reports were published in 1948. The titles were
Nursing for the Future, authored by Esther Lucille Brown,
Ph.D. and *A Program for the Nursing Profession*, authored by
the Committee on the Function of Nursing, Eli Ginzberg,
Chairman.(1)(2) A report was published in 1959 titled
Community College Education for Nursing, authored by
Mildred Montag.(3) This report is so important in telling
the story of American nursing that it will be removed from
the present context and discussed in the next chapter. In
1962 the Surgeon General's Consultant Group on Nursing
published a report titled *Toward Quality Nursing*.(4) In 1970,
the Report of the National Commission on Nursing and
Nursing Education was published under the title *Abstract
for Action*.(5)

Nursing for the Future, or the Brown Report, was
sponsored by the Carnegie Corporation and the Russell
Sage Foundation. This report was essentially a restatement
of the Goldmark Report and the Report of the Committee
on the Grading of Nursing Schools that were published
in the 1920s. Brown presented a narrative with little
documentation regarding sources of information. However,
one nurse historian was positively impressed.

Due to its incandescent quality, intrinsic merit, and the enthusiasm with which its sale was promoted by the profession, the distribution of the Brown report exceeded that of any other social study known to Dr. Brown.(6)

The report essentially advocated the official party line: move nursing education into the collegiate setting.

A Program for the Nursing Profession, or the Ginsberg Report, was of a different quality. There was less discussion of the nurse as victim, and the report did not concentrate on past wrongs perpetrated on American nursing. The major focus was the role of nurses in solving their enduring problems. The Ginsberg Report took the nursing establishment to task on a number of issues, such as lack of support for the practical nurse.

Past relations between the professional and practical nurse give cause for serious concern. The responsible leadership that the situation demanded of professional nurses has seldom been in evidence. In general, leaders of the nursing profession have pursued a defensive exclusionist policy, devoting their efforts to protecting their own domain and displaying much hostility and little concern for those who remain outside.(7)

This was direct and to the point. The Ginsberg Report also addressed the subsidiary worker in relation to the cost of nursing care delivery in the hospital. Keep in mind this report was published in 1948. The military model of nursing care delivery had been highly successful, and the subsidiary worker was a major player in the success of that model. This reality was still fresh in the minds of many. However, the nursing establishment still did not buy into the subsidiary worker concept, and the Ginzberg Report pointed to this fact in the following statement.

> Moreover, as nurses, they were unconcerned about the waste of personnel resources entailed by the exclusive use of highly trained professional personnel for all nursing care.(8)

Ginzberg was correct. The cost of delivering nursing care in the hospital setting was not a concern for the nursing establishment. The Ginsberg Report of 1948 echoed the Goldmark Report of 1922. Both reports supported subsidiary workers and two formats for nursing education and practice. The distinction was the nature of the two formats.

The Goldmark Report supported the hospital as the training site for nurses in the acute care in-patient setting. The college setting should be utilized for training the educators, supervisors and public health nurses. The Ginsberg Report proposed nursing functions be divided among professional and practical nurses. The professional nurse would complete a four-year course in a college or university setting. The practical nurse would complete a nine- to twelve-month course in a school of practical or vocational nursing. The proposal was a two-tiered system that was essentially already in place. Some of the infrastructure was available in the form of existing practical nurse training programs.

The question of maintaining the hospital three-year diploma program was already under increased scrutiny.

The situation was ripe for change, and the stage was set for implementation. Moving nursing education from the hospital into the university and creating additional practical nurse training programs was a reasonable fix for what was ailing American nursing. It failed to happen for three reasons. First, the nursing establishment would not support a two-tiered system in which the practical nurse assumed an integral role. Second, the two-year associate degree nursing educational program was introduce by Mildred Montag of Teachers College, Columbia University. Montag's endeavor would take educational focus and potential students away from the four-year nursing program. Third, the nursing establishment was not held accountable to implement needed changes within their purview. An empowered oversight body to direct change in the best interests of both American nursing and American society was not a reality in 1948. Such an entity remains absent to this very day.

In 1961 the perennial nursing shortage was particularly acute. The federal government sought a role in providing adequate nursing services for the nation.(9) The Surgeon General of the Public Health Service appointed a group comprised mostly of doctors (MDs) and nurses (RNs). Their formal title was the Surgeon General's Consultant Group on Nursing. In 1962, they issued a report titled *Toward Quality in Nursing.* Their very first recommendation was the following:

A study should be made of the present system of nursing education in relation to the responsibilities and skill levels required for high quality patient care. This study should be started immediately so that nursing education programs can benefit as soon as possible from the findings. Funds for such a study should be obtained from private and government sources.(10)

Once again, a recommendation for another study. Once again, a sense of foreboding regarding the educational process in nursing as demonstrated by the following:

The present educational structure for the training of nurses lacks system, order and coherence. There is no clear differentiation as to the levels of responsibility for which the graduates of each type of program are prepared.(11)

The major accomplishment of the consultant group was the formation of the National Commission for the Study of Nursing and Nursing Education. The report of this group was published in 1970 under the title *Abstract for Action*. This was the most prescriptive of the reports, and it caused great anxiety and some anger within the nursing establishment. Unfortunately and as usual, the anxiety and anger did not foster any significant change.

The director and author of the report was Jerome Lysaught, a professor of education at the University of Rochester. The members of the commission were mainly educators. Their presence and influence is easily recognized via the emphasis on process and detail in the final report.

The report was comprehensive. The first several chapters of the document are a review of American nursing history, the periodic nursing shortages, the relationship between nursing and other disciplines, nursing educational programs, professional nursing organizations, and the American healthcare scene. Findings and recommendations are specified in three chapters titled "Nursing Roles and Functions," "Nursing Education," and "Nursing Careers." Each chapter has seventeen to twenty-two recommendations and most of these have a sub-set of recommendations. The recommendations are condensed into four priorities. The report concludes with three central recommendations. Needless to say, it is a difficult read. However, there are some clear and pertinent statements that warranted consideration at the time of publication and retrospectively for the purposes of this narrative.

> Since 1923 there has been a succession of studies, inquiries and investigations into nursing in the United States. These studies have had limited impact on the profession itself and on related institutions and healthcare groups. This inaction has stemmed in large measure from inertia. In addition, some antagonism toward change has been generated among the groups that make up the health professions.(12)

The statement confirmed what everyone knew— American nursing was a well-studied entity. The statement also indicates a growing weariness with the resistance to change demonstrated by nursing specifically and the healthcare sector in general. The report offers another disconcerting observation.

> The long history of national nursing studies, dating back to 1922, is ample evidence that the profession alone cannot be expected to effect the recommendations

enunciated for its improvement. Nursing must have the sympathy and help of the other professions, the administrators of health facilities and the general public.(13)

A national commission informed American nursing and the general public that nursing was not capable of effecting needed changes required for success in the remainder of the twentieth century. Surprisingly, this observation did not stir action for change within the nursing establishment. However, *Abstract for Action* repeated a familiar refrain that did elicit a response from the nursing establishment. Specifically, a proposal was made that two essentially related but different career patterns should be developed for nursing practice.

a. One career pattern (episodic) would emphasize nursing practice that is essentially curative and restorative, generally acute or chronic in nature, and most frequently provided in the setting of the hospital or in-patient facility.

b. The second career pattern (distributive) would emphasize the nursing practice that is designed essentially for health maintenance and disease prevention, generally continuous in nature, seldom acute, and most frequently operative in the community or in newly developing institutional settings.(14)

Of all the studies/reports of the era, *Abstract for Action* at least ruffled a few nursing feathers. Noted nurse historian Teresa Christy, a prominent member of the nursing establishment and two colleagues, wrote a stinging article titled, "An Appraisal of an Abstract for Action."(15) She lashed out at the author as well as the content. She cited failure to use primary sources. She believed the Commission demonstrated a bias favorable toward hospitals as educational institutions. She questioned research methods utilized to conduct and summarize the study. She was incensed by improper documentation of historical data.

> The report is erroneous in its historical citation and less than precise in its scholarship. Some readers may say the point made is minor but we believe it illustrates the lack of attention to careful detail evident throughout the entire document.(16)

Christy, the NLN, and the nursing establishment in general failed to address the issues raised in this report. However, there was no ambiguity regarding their rejection of the recommendations concerning episodic and distributive career pathways for nursing practice. Christy described the recommendations as drastic and divisive and did not prepare the nurse to care for the whole individual. She elaborated on the obvious. "They seem to promote a dichotomy between care in different settings as well as in the kinds of knowledge needed to meet the nursing needs of people."(17) Her statement described the essence of the basic changes needed in nursing and she cannot contain her incredulousness.

Christy was not alone in her disinclination. The NLN, supposedly the premier organization for nursing education in the United States, made a response that mimicked

Christy's attention to process rather than substance. In general the NLN response was one of requesting further clarification of issues and recommending rephrasing of statements. The NLN never made a formal response regarding the two career pathways and did not take a stand on the issue.(18)

Again, the nursing establishment ignored the important issues of the day. This was the most definitive report of the century. Or was it just too definitive? The title, *Abstract for Action,* was indicative of a blueprint to overcome obstacles that plagued American nursing. The report was detailed and exhaustive. In retrospect, it may have been just too broad an endeavor and the essentials such as the episodic and distributive career pathways were lost in the numerous findings and recommendations. There would be additional reports, but none would rise to the level of comprehensiveness of *Abstract for Action.*

The Commission recommended the establishment of a national joint practice commission between medicine (AMA) and nursing (ANA). The purpose was to examine the congruent roles of physician and nurse in providing quality health care.(19) This recommendation became a reality in 1972 in the form of the National Joint Practice Committee. The Committee remained in existence until 1981 when, without explanation, the AMA withdrew from the arrangement. It is implied in some literature the nursing membership was agitating for an independent role in the provision of patient care. The Commission recommended state licensure laws require periodic review of the nurse's qualifications as a requisite for licensure renewal.(20) Indeed, some states passed laws specifying continuing education units as a requisite for license renewal. A recommendation was made that each state have a master planning committee that would take nursing education under its purview. The rationale for this recommendation was "because education is an area reserved to the states" and "local conditions are important ingredients in the planning and timing of change." According to the 1973 publication *From Abstract into Action,* twenty-six states created master planning committees. "Progress and pace of activity are varied; however, the groundswell of involvement and planning for action is clearly observable."(21) State master planning committees did not become a creative driving force in American nursing. This recommendation was illogical. Fifty master planning committees were not needed by American nursing or American society.

A general theme is discernible in the studies under discussion. The commonality is the two-pronged approach to nursing practice and/or nursing education. Goldmark differentiated between the hospital-trained nurse and the university-educated nurse educator, nurse administrator, and public health nurse. Ginzberg recommended the university-trained professional nurse and the vocationally trained, practical nurse. Lysaught recommended episodic and distributive career pathways. Specifics differed according to author and time frame. However, there was a general message. Narrow the focus of nursing practice and educate accordingly.

The nursing establishment failed to heed this very good advice, and there was a reason for their recalcitrance. As discussed in the previous chapter and from the nursing establishment's perspective, it was a control issue. If the two-pronged approach was implemented, the nursing establishment would be linked permanently and exclusively to those nurses educated in the college setting and/or working in community-based programs, public health agencies, nursing administration and education. Their sphere of influence would be reduced—substantially.

Lysaught, as director of the Commission for the Study of Nursing and Nursing Education, published three other treatises in conjunction with the original *Abstract for Action*. *From Abstract into Action* was published in 1973, and *Action in Nursing* was published in 1974. *Abstract in Affirmation* was published in 1981.(22, 23, 24) He envisioned "a continuing agency that would persevere for some years to accomplish the Commission's recommendations." He further elaborated that such an agency "could be our one assurance that the year 2000 would not see just one more link in the long chain of nursing studies that are filled with sound and fury—signifying nothing."(25)

The continuing agency did not become a reality. However, the W.K. Kellogg Foundation, the ANA, and the NLN contributed financial support allowing an additional three years of life for the Commission. Lysaught was a prolific writer regarding the problems of American nursing. He demonstrated a keen awareness of the failure of the nursing establishment to respond to pressing issues of the day. Lysaught 's concept of a continuing agency was a step in the right direction. However, it would have been advisory or consultative in nature. The real need was and remains an official and centralized planning agency with authority to implement needed changes in nursing practice and nursing education. This will be discussed in detail in a subsequent chapter.

Throughout the years, considerable time, effort and money has been expended on behalf of American nursing in an effort to stabilize this would-be profession. The nursing establishment failed to buy into the many solid recommendations made in the numerous reports. Their tenacious belief that nursing was a profession and the lack of a centralized empowered entity to serve in an oversight capacity allowed the recalcitrance of the establishment to prevail. To make matters even more inexplicable, Mildred Montag came forward with a two-year community college nursing program. The identity and some would say the integrity of American nursing education was changed forever by an idea actualized by this one woman. Many in the nursing establishment supported Montag. Others stood by and did nothing.

References

1. Brown, Esther Lucille. *Nursing for the Future.* New York: Russell Sage Foundation. 1948.
2. Committee on the Function of Nursing. *A Program for the Nursing Profession.* New York: Macmillan Company. 1948.
3. Montag Mildred. *Community College Education for Nursing.* McGraw-Hill Book Company Inc. 1959.
4. Surgeon General's Consultant Group on Nursing. *Toward Quality in Nursing.* U.S. Department of Health, Education and Welfare. 1962.
5. The National Commission for the Study of Nursing and Nursing Education. *An Abstract for Action.* Jerome P. Lysaught, Director. New York: McGraw-Hill Company. 1970.

6. Roberts, Mary. *American Nursing*. New York: The Macmillan Company. 1954. pg. 516.

7. Committee on the Function of Nursing. pg. 72.

8. *ibid.*

9. Surgeon General's Consultant Group on Nursing. pg. xiii.

10. *ibid.* pg. 55–56.

11. *ibid.* pg. 13.

12. The National Commission for the Study of Nursing and Nursing Education. pg. 21.

13. *ibid.* pg. 151.

14. *ibid.* pg. 91.

15. Christy, Teresa. Muriel A. Polin and Julie Hover. "An Appraisal of an Abstract for Action." *American Journal of Nursing*. August, 1971. pg. 1574-1581.

16. *ibid.* pg. 1575.

17. *ibid.* pg. 1579–1580.

18. National League of Nursing. " Report of the Task Force to Study the Implications of the Recommendations Presented in An Abstract for Action." *Nursing Outlook*. Volume 21. #2. (February 1973).

19. *Abstract for Action.* pg. 89.

20. *ibid.* pg. 142.

21. Lysaught, Jerome P. *From Abstract into Action.* New York: McGraw-Hill Book Company. 1973. pg. 153–55.

22. *ibid.* pg.

23. Lysaught, Jerome P., editor. *Action in Nursing.* New York: McGraw-Hill Company. 1974.

24. Lysaught, Jerome P. *Abstract in Affirmation.* New York: McGraw Hill Book Company. 1981.

25. *Abstract for Action.* pg. 163.

9

MILDRED'S MISCONCEPTION

Modern American nursing and Teachers College, Columbia University, have a long historical association. It commenced in 1899 when Hampton-Robb and Dean Russell made the study of nursing a junior contender In the academic world. The first doctoral program for nurses, an Ed.D. in nursing education, was established in the early 1920s.(1) Other graduate nursing programs have surpassed the institution in the study of nursing practice. However, Teachers College has never ceased being a major influence in nursing education. Perhaps the greatest influence was realized via the inextricable association of Teachers College, Mildred Montag, and the two-year associate degree nursing educational program. The results of this association had the most significant impact on modern American nursing since the late nineteenth century endeavors of the early lady reformers at Bellevue. In 1999, the Nursing Education

Alumni Association held a centennial celebration. In the *Commemorative Report*, they came forward with the phrase "Celebrating a Century of Influence." As the saying goes, "truer words were never spoken."

The historical time frame is the immediate post WWII era. A great deal was happening in terms of hospitals, nursing, and education in general. The Hospital Survey and Construction Act of 1946 (Hill-Burton Act) significantly increased the number of hospital beds throughout the United States. An increasing number of Americans had hospital insurance, thus increasing access to hospital care. Additional hospital beds and additional patients called for additional nurses. However, there was also a general decline in nursing school enrollments. Many of the military nurses returned to civilian life, married, stayed home, and raised children. More young women were now going to college in preparation for a variety of careers other than teaching and nursing. There was also the relatively new phenomenon known as the two-year junior/community college.

Thus began a frantic attempt to deal with another nursing shortage. At mid-point in the twentieth century, the nation needed nurses. Mildred Montag, a nurse, utilizing the junior/community college system, would give the nation what she conceived the nation needed. She would educate a new type of nurse and do it in two academic years. She would call this individual a nursing technician. However, Montag omitted an important preliminary step. She failed to consult the hospital industry regarding the desire or need for a new vaguely defined type of nurse. This was the basis of Mildred's misconception.

Montag was awarded an Ed.D. from Teachers College, Columbia University in 1950. In 1951, she published a book titled *Education of Nursing Technicians*.(2) The book was based on her doctoral dissertation. In 1952, the Institute for Nursing Research at Teachers College was established. In 1954, under the aegis of the Institute, the Cooperative Research Project in Junior and Community College Education for Nursing was inaugurated. The project director was Montag. She was given the opportunity of a lifetime. She would implement her doctoral dissertation.

Montag's basic assertion regarding her proposed program had, in part, a familiar resonance. Like many prewar commission reports, Montag called for two levels of nursing practice, one professional and one technical in nature. The professional nurse would be the four-year baccalaureate degree nurse. The technical nurse would be the two-year associate degree nurse. She did not address the fact the three-year hospital diploma program still supplied the majority of nursing school graduates in the United States. Also, she did not address the fact that practical nursing programs were increasing in number throughout the nation and their graduates were establishing a successful presence in the hospital setting.

At mid-twentieth century and as a consequence of Mildred's misconception, American nursing education consisted of a four-year college nursing program, a three-year hospital diploma program, a one-year vocational school program, and Montag's technical two-year junior/community college program. This unique and multifaceted approach to American nursing education soon created a significant level of consternation within nursing circles.

"Would the real nurse please stand up?" became a familiar and sometimes sarcastic refrain.

And then there was the licensure issue. At the initiation of her project, Montag successfully negotiated with individual state boards of nursing to allow the two-year associate degree graduate to take the RN licensure examination. The American nursing scene would now have graduates of four-year baccalaureate programs, three-year hospital diploma programs, and two-year associate degree programs taking the same licensure examination for status as an RN. The enigmatic Montag claimed there was an essential difference between the four-year baccalaureate graduate and her two-year technical graduate. However, she claimed no such difference when it came to licensure of these individuals. This state of affairs represented incongruity at its best. This inconsistency in the education and licensing of the American nurse was a reality that did not seem to bother the nursing establishment or state boards of nursing. Why this was tolerated will be discussed in a later chapter.

Where did the technician idea originate? The term came from the field of engineering. However, it was brought to the nursing scene by Esther Lucille Brown of *Nursing for the Future* fame. In her treatise, Brown wrote a chapter titled, "Differentiation of Nursing Service According to Function." In the chapter, there was a segment titled "Engineering an Example of Differentiated Functions." The term "engineering technician" is used to describe different levels of practice within the field of engineering. She said the following in reference to the education of engineering technicians.

The course of study is generally two years in length. All curricula are more distinctly vocational than are the four-year engineering colleges.(3)

Thus, the concept of technician was borrowed from the engineering domain. Montag coined the title "nurse technician." "The name nursing technician is suggested as the name of the new worker."(4) Also, the term "technician" was consistent with the evolving community college movement, which identified many of their programs as technical or semi-professional in nature.(5) Armed with a borrowed concept and a new nursing title, Montag proceeded with her demonstration project aimed at producing a technical nurse.

Seven junior/community colleges and one hospital school of nursing were selected for the Cooperative Research Project (Fairleigh Dickinson University in Rutherford, New Jersey; Henry Ford Community College in Dearborn, Michigan; Orange County Community College in Middletown, New York; Pasadena City College in Pasadena, California; Virginia Intermont College in Bristol, Virginia; Virginia State College in Norfork, Virginia; Weber College in Ogden, Utah; and Monmouth Memorial Hospital in Long Branch, New Jersey).

The reasons given for inclusion of a hospital school of nursing are vague at best. Curriculum content and format, clinical experience, and length of program were the major variables that distinguished the project program from the traditional hospital three-year program. In terms of curriculum, the project program had general academic and nursing courses presented in the semester credit-hour format typical of college level courses. In contrast, hospital programs offered condensed science courses at the beginning of the program and disease-oriented clinical courses distributed throughout the calendar year.

In terms of clinical experience, the project program was characterized by a highly structured learning environment. The student entered the clinical environment with a specific learning objective, i.e., care for a diabetic patient requiring foot care. There was a pre-conference, during which students and instructor discussed the day's learning objectives. The student would then enter the clinical area and provide nursing care to a designated patient. Once the day's clinical objectives were accomplished, the student retreated from the clinical area and attended a post-conference with the instructor and other students. The purpose of this conference was to review the day's learning experience and correlate theoretical concepts learned in the classroom with the clinical experience.

The number of hours spent in the clinical area was not the focus. The focus was the accomplishment of specific learning objectives. Identifying and implementing the student's learning objectives was the driving force of the project program. In contrast, "learn by doing" and "come what may" are the phrases best describing the driving force of student learning experiences in hospital programs. Also, the eight-hour day was common in hospital programs. The project program was usually two academic years and one summer session in length. The hospital program was three calendar years. The project program did not rely on repetition as a learning tool. In contrast, repetition was the hallmark of the hospital program.

Montag was not impressed with the utilization of repetition as a learning tool. The following statement by Montag is in reference to the project program and learning by repetition.

> ...is not hampered by needless repetition, nor is it diluted by extraneous activities desirable for doing the work of the hospital but not conducive to learning by the student.(6)

The elimination of repetition as a tool of learning allowed the project program to be completed in less time. This of course was an attractive feature to prospective students. However, the elimination of repetition as a learning tool also curtailed the student's exposure to the clinical area. This in turn promoted a major problem. The lack of clinical experience in their nursing educational program is the underlying source of work anxiety expressed by many two-year associate degree graduate nurses starting a career in the in-patient setting. Technical skills, proficiency, and self-confidence come together as a whole only with practice. This was true in the 1950s and remains true today.

Montag's Cooperative Research project demonstrated that a basic nursing educational program could be integrated into a community/junior college system. Graduates of these programs could earn an associate degree in nursing and could pass the RN licensure examination. However, problems soon developed for employers of graduates of the two-year nursing program. The employers soon realized the consequences of the limited clinical experience afforded these students: they were simply not prepared to assume the position of beginning graduate nurse. Employers soon acquiesced to the reality the necessary skills would only be obtained via extensive on-the-job training.

Most graduates of the associate degree nursing programs would eventually obtain the skills needed to function as a beginning graduate nurse. It was estimated novice status for these graduates could extend to two years.(7) A basic tenet of the associate degree program is that students, upon graduation, are prepared to *become* competent nurses rather than *be* competent.(8) According to the Montag model, it was the employer's responsibility to develop a fully competent nurse. The employer was to provide the technical nurse with the finishing touches consistent with clinical experience of the three-year hospital diploma program. This was the message sent to hospital administrators and directors of nursing in the 1950s and 1960s. However, hospital administrators and directors of nursing had a different perspective on the issue. They were accustomed to dealing with three-year hospital apprentice trained nurses. These nurses made an easy transition to graduate nurse/new employee status. Consequently, administrators of that era did not take easily to the dictate that associate degree graduates required extensive training at hospital expense. It appeared to some all Montag accomplished with her new program was reduction of time spent in gaining clinical experience. It seemed to many she mandated the traditional third-year of the hospital diploma apprenticeship program back to the employer, only now the employer was paying a salary to the neophyte nurse.

Associate degree nursing programs proliferated throughout the 1960s and 1970s, as did the community college system. Eventually the programs outnumbered baccalaureate and hospital nursing programs. It was obvious to all concerned that the programs were here to stay, as were some vexing problems for the nursing establishment. Operationally defining the term "technical nurse" became a major issue. Montag's definition did not fit the reality of the work situation. The following statement by Montag is her attempt to explain the difference between the professional and technical nurse. It was statements such as the following that greatly concerned directors of nursing in the hospital industry.

> There are two basic premises on which the associate degree program was developed: 1) that the functions of nursing can and should be differentiated, and 2) that these functions lie along a continuum, with professional at one end and technical at the other. At one point on the continuum, of course, the functions meet, and the technician's role comes close to that of the professional. But that does not mean that the technician is a professional or that the professional is a technician. If the functions can be differentiated, then it follows that the two kinds of workers should be prepared differently, for the two kinds of functions— hence two programs, one professional and one technical.(9)

The nurse with technical preparation would be prepared to do, with supervision, the bulk of nursing care given to patients. It is obvious that they should not be expected to assume responsibility for, or to carry out, treatments and care that require skill and judgment beyond the limits of their training. The technically trained nurse would then perform functions requiring skill and judgment beyond that of the aide but less than that of the nurse with professional preparation.(10)

Obviously, Montag could not operationally describe the technical nurse at the patient care level. In 1976, an experienced director of nursing explained why this was not possible. She did not resort to ambiguity or equivocation when she wrote the following:

Clearly, the difficulties with this concept begin at the point at which these assumptions touch down on actual nurse-patient interactions. Unfortunately, the patient does not present his needs in neat bundles that can be clearly identified as chiefly technical or professional, but rather they are emitted in unsorted, intermingled, unpredictable packages which must be dealt with by the practitioner who is present with the patient at the particular time.(11)

The separation of the technical from the professional function is a theoretical construct that simply does not stand the test of practice.(12)

Montag's misconception was a major blunder. This in turn caused friction between nurse educators and directors of nursing in hospital settings. It became a blame game. Nurse educators were told they did not know how to train nurses. Directors of nursing were told they did not know how to utilize the nurse technician in the clinical situation.

In time, the term "technical nurse" was put aside as not workable. New rhetoric was used in an attempt to provide some consistency in describing characteristics of the different types of educationally prepared nurses with the initials RN. The terms "competencies" and "differentiated practice" came on the scene. Again, even with these new terms, ambiguity remained in full force. At the operational level, i.e., the patient's bedside, it was not possible to demonstrate an essential difference between the graduates of different types of programs. In reference to all this confusion the Surgeon General of the United States referred to nursing as "a deeply troubled profession."(13)

Today the majority of American nurses are educated at the community college level and earn an associate degree in nursing. They are the largest segment of nurses holding the title RN, the title traditionally accepted as the designation of the professional nurse. The majority of nurses in the United States lack what is considered a professional education. Hampton-Robb and Nutting would certainly be disappointed. In 1899, at Teachers College, they attempted the professionalization of American nursing via the educational route. In 1957, at Teachers College, Montag solidified the deprofessionalization of American nursing via the educational route.

The Brown Report, *Nursing for the Future*, and the Ginzberg Report, *A Program for the Nursing Profession*, recommended the upgrading of practical nurse education. Some of Montag's nurse contemporaries recommended the upgrading of practical nurse education via the associate degree program. This was a logical proposal. It was consistent with the vocational orientation of community college education. Also, some of Montag's contemporaries warned that implementation of the nurse technician concept was not in the best interests of nursing. Lulu K. Wolf Hassenplug was one such person.

> I tried unsuccessfully to get the name of these programs changed to vocational nurse programs so that we would eventually have only two programs for nursing when the diploma schools were discontinued, but I lost the battle to Louise McManus. Who didn't lose when arguing with Louise? Now we have associate and baccalaureate degree programs preparing nurses for the same license to practice, and this continues to create more problems than it solves.(14)

Montag and colleagues at Teachers College ignored their contemporaries. R. Louise McManus was the director, Division of Nursing Education at Teachers College and Montag's boss at the time of the Cooperative Research Project. She was a powerful figure in American nursing. An air of arrogance is evident in the following statement by McManus.

> As soon as word got about that Teachers College was about to start experimentation in registered nurse preparation in two years, protests poured in from nurse educators in diploma schools and baccalaureate

programs alike and from nursing leaders at the League headquarters. Proceeding with our plan would sell nursing down the river, we were told. I defended both the need and the university's right and responsibility to carry on research, turned deaf ears to their protests, and continued plans to get under way.(15)

In retrospect, McManus, Montag, et. al., accomplished quite a feat. They provided the hospital industry with a new type of graduate nurse, albeit one with extended learning needs. They confused everyone regarding the nature and intent of the various nursing educational programs. They confounded the purpose of licensing laws for nurses, at least in the mind of any logical person. They established the groundwork for warfare between nurse educators of the different types of nursing educational programs. Finally, they did irreparable harm by pitting nurses against each other in defense of their educational preparation. No wonder American nursing never cultivated the dynamic cohesiveness necessary to act and speak as one.

How and why were a few nurse educators able to have such a major impact on American nursing? There is no indication of any type of power play with any official government agency. Montag make it quite clear she dealt only with state boards of nursing who looked favorably on her two-year program.(16) In fact, why were the state boards of nursing, overseers of the licensing function, so amenable to the two-year program? This question is not asked nor answered in the nursing literature. Perhaps Montag and McManus exerted an arrogance of influence consistent with their association with Teachers College. Perhaps Eleanor C. Lambersten, a nursing educator and Teachers College functionary explained the situation when she stated the following:

> Teachers College was viewed by everyone as the place to receive a degree. The world greats in nursing education were, or had been, on the faculty. The alumni were in power positions.(17)

State boards of nursing are official agencies with obligations to the citizenry. Nursing educators are overseers of the academic integrity of nursing educational programs. Montag was a woman with an idea. How and why was Montag's proposal allowed to proceed and consume the identity of American nursing? The answer has roots in the lack of an empowered oversight group. Montag answered only to McManus. The two prominent nursing organizations of the day, the ANA and NLN, responded after the fact and then essentially accommodated the program. Regardless, they were powerless to halt the program at inception. The women from Teachers College changed the very countenance of American nursing, and they did it their way. How? There simply was no one to stop them!

References

1. Donahue, Patricia M. *Nursing the Finest Art.* St. Louis: C.V. Mosby Company. 1985. pg. 456.
2. Montag, Mildred L. *The Education of Nursing Technicians.* New York: G.P. Putnam and Sons. 1951.

3. Brown, Esther Lucille. *Nursing for the Future*. New York: Russell Sage Foundation. 1948. pg. 63–66.

4. Montag. *The Education of Nursing Technicians*. pg. 135.

5. Haase, Patricia T. *The Origins and Rise of Associate Degree Nursing Education*. Durham: Duke University Press. 1990. pg. 98.

6. Montag, Mildred. L. *Community College Education for Nursing*. New York: McGraw-Hill Book Company, Inc. 1959. pg. 95.

7. Hass. pg. 143.

8. Montag. *Community College Education for Nursing*. pg. 4.

9. Montag. Mildred L. "Looking Back: Associate Degree Education in Perspective." *Nursing Outlook*. April, 1980. pg. 249.

10. Montag. *The Education of Nursing Technicians*. pg. 71.

11. McClure, Margaret. "Can We Bring Order Out of the Chaos of Nursing Education." *American Journal of Nursing*. January, 1976. pg. 101.

12. *ibid*. pg. 101.

13. "The Surgeon General Looks at Nursing." *American Journal of Nursing*. January, 1967. pg. 64.

14. Safier, Gwendolyn. *Contemporary American Leaders in Nursing*. New York: McGraw-Hill Books. 1977. pg. 42.

15. *ibid*. pg. 200.

16. Montag. *Community College Education for Nurses*. pg. 32.

17. Safier. pg. 42.

10

THE '60S, THE '70S, AND THE PROFESSIONAL ISSUE

In 1945, a new set of criteria was put forth to identify a profession. In comparison to the Flexner criteria of 1915, these new criteria were more accommodating to the nursing cause. Genevieve and Roy Bixler, both with the Ed.D. credential from Columbia University, published an article in the *American Journal of Nursing*. The title was "The Professional Status of Nursing." (1) The Bixlers outlined seven criteria they considered necessary for professional standing.

1. There is a well defined and well organized body of specialized knowledge.

2. A profession utilizes the scientific method.

3. The education of professionals takes place in institutions of higher learning.

4. A profession applies its body of knowledge in services vital to human and social welfare.

5. A profession functions autonomously in the control of professional activity.

6. A profession attracts individuals of intellectual and personal qualities who put service above personal gain and view their occupation as a life work.

7. A profession compensates its practitioners by providing freedom of action, opportunity for continuous professional growth and economic security.

What was the Bixlers' conclusion regarding the professional status of nursing? They never put forth a definitive answer.

The reader of the article might conclude nursing had made progress toward professional status but had not yet arrived on the professional scene. In 1959, the Bixlers wrote a progress report.(2) Again, the reader might conclude progress had been made but nursing had not yet arrived. In the 1960s and 1970s, the nursing establishment engaged in a frenzy of academic activity aimed at meeting the professional criteria identified by the Bixlers. Development of a theory of nursing, conducting nursing research, graduate education for nurses, and autonomy in practice all became prominent issues. However, Bixler Criterion number three—education for professionals takes place in institutions of higher learning—was special. This was a criterion the nursing establishment believed they most certainly could implement.

The ANA was so confident about meeting this criterion the organization actually took a stand on the subject and published a position paper. Time would demonstrate the organization made a fateful decision. The position paper would divide American nurses. "The division was deep, and it boded ill for nursing as a whole."(3)

The '60s and '70s were watershed decades for American nursing. Discussion concerning the professional status issue reached a pinnacle and even received a new label. It became known as "entry into practice" issue. The general theme of professional status for nurses became specific. The focus now was who could claim the title "professional nurse" and how should that person be educated. The ANA not only published a paper that defined professional nursing education but attempted to convince state legislatures that education for professional nursing should be defined by state law. As a result of these two initiatives the ANA alienated multiple segments of their own constituency. Along the way nurse educators and community supporters of associate degree nursing programs developed a "don't tread on me" attitude. By the conclusion of the 1970s, the balkanization of American nursing was complete.

The American Nurses Association Position Paper on Education for Nursing represents a failure and public humiliation for American nursing. Known in nursing circles as the Position Paper, it was published in the December 1965 issue of the *American Journal of Nursing*. (4) The purpose of the Position Paper was to promote the placement of all nursing education into two- or four-year college programs. Only graduates of baccalaureate degree programs would qualify for the title professional nurse.

The ANA made several strategic errors. They acted on a false assumption. They assumed that mandating changes at the academic level would automatically effect desired changes and acceptance within all of nursing. They ignored the potential social and psychological impact for nurses without baccalaureate degrees who considered themselves professional nurses, i.e., the hospital diploma graduate. The real world of state licensing laws was completely ignored. These mistakes, acting in a vacuum, were similar to those made by Montag in implementing the associate degree program. The ANA, supposedly the national organization for all nurses, took a major stand that essentially ignored the realities of the day and discriminated against the majority of their members. The majority of their constituents were nurses without baccalaureate degrees.

Nurses in the academic sector herald the Position Paper as the answer to the problems noted in the numerous reports of previous years. Directors of nursing, particularly in the hospital situation, were apprehensive. There were serious implications for the hospital nursing organization. It was 1965, and the majority of the nation's nurses were still three-year hospital diploma graduates. Included in this group were the supervisors and head nurses, vital players in any nursing organization. Hospital diploma school graduates considered themselves the bulwark of the ANA, and they considered themselves professionals. They were stunned and angered by the action of their national organization. The response from the associate degree sector was interesting. Graduates of these programs were still relatively new on the scene. They did not overtly covet the title of professional nurse. These nurses were more concerned with maintaining the state designated title of RN.

Exactly what did the Position Paper say to nurses and the American public?

The narrative in general was not contentious. Minus some specific statements, the Position Paper would have been acceptable to most nurses. It was the following statements that set in motion much of the future unrest within American nursing.

> ...minimum preparation for beginning professional nursing practice at the present time should be baccalaureate degree education in nursing.

> ...minimum preparation for beginning technical nursing practice at the present time should be associate degree education in nursing.

> ...the nursing profession ... [to] systematically work to facilitate the replacement of programs for practical nursing with programs for beginning technical nursing practice in junior and community colleges.(5)

Simply stated, only graduates of four-year baccalaureate programs would be considered professional nurses; graduates of two-year associate degree programs would be the technical non-professional nurse; practical nursing programs would go out of business.

These were highly charged statements in view of a few facts. The stand taken toward practical nursing programs was not in concert with that of the federal government. The latter was providing practical nursing programs with permanent financial aid, authorized by the 1963 Vocational Education Act. The Position Paper did not address state licensing laws governing the RN and LPN titles. The future status of the hospital diploma nurse was not even mentioned. Representatives of the largest segment of the nurse population of the day were completely ignored. (It should be noted that regardless of the Position Paper, the future of hospital diploma programs was not promising. By the 1960s these programs were becoming too expensive to operate. Student nurses were no longer an integral part of hospital staffing, which meant they were no longer a financial asset. Hospital diploma programs went into rapid decline. By 1975, they represented less than a third of all nursing educational programs.)(6) By the year 2000, few diploma programs remained in existence and the two-year associate degree program had surpassed in number the four-year baccalaureate degree program. By the year 2000, American nursing was comprised mainly of a technically educated workforce.

The major tenet of the 1965 Position Paper, education for professional nursing practice should take place at the baccalaureate degree level, did not gain the expected momentum. The majority of potential students selected the two-year associate degree nursing program. Something had to be done to get back on course. An ANA sponsored conference was held in February 1978, and a number of resolutions were forthcoming. One in particular read as follows:

That the ANA ensure two categories of nursing practice to be identified and titled by 1980, that by 1985, the minimum preparation for entry into professional nursing practice be the baccalaureate in nursing.(7)

This course correction was known as the 1985 Proposal. However, the ANA specifically and the nursing establishment in general continued to ignore a basic fact of life. Only the individual states via their licensing laws could ensure the designation of professional and technical nurse. Like the ANA Position Paper proposals, the 1985 Proposal did not gain momentum.

The ANA House of Delegates adopted yet another proposal. It read as follows:

The ANA House of Delegates agreed to establish the goal that the baccalaureate for professional nursing practice be implemented in

5% of the states by 1986
15% of the states by 1988
50% of the states by 1992
100%f the states by 1995.(8)

This proposal at least acknowledged that significant work had to be accomplished at the state level and it just might take some time. However, with very few exceptions, states would not even consider such designations. The ANA 1965 Position Paper on Nursing Education and the 1985 Proposal did not become reality.

Eventually the ANA lost interest with the "entry into practice" issue and became a serious participant in the labor movement. The organization was now a bargaining agent for RNs from all three basic nursing educational programs. Practically speaking, it was simply not in the organization's best interests to focus on an issue that favored only one segment of the organization's membership. During this time frame, the early 1980s, there were 1,432 educational programs preparing student nurses to take the RN licensing examination. There were 288 hospital diploma programs, 742 associate degree programs, and 402 baccalaureate degree programs.(9)

However, there were a few ANA foot soldiers at the state level who attempted to implement the national organization's 1985 proposal. New York led the way. New York State Nurses Association's (NYSNA) 1985 Proposal would require a baccalaureate degree in nursing for licensure as a professional nurse and an associate degree in nursing for licensure as a practical nurse. These new requirements would not apply to any individual with a license issued prior to 1984.(10)

The New York proposal differed from the 1965 ANA Proposal. It differentiated according to professional and practical nursing rather than professional and technical nursing. The New York Proposal was in accordance with the Brown and Ginzberg reports of previous decades. However, New York nurses remained divided regarding the issue, and it became evident compromise was not an option. Many reasons were offered for failure to reach an agreement. There was the cost issue. Educating all professional nurses in four-year college programs would be very expensive if not prohibitive. The tax-payer would eventually be called upon to assume the financial burden. Four-year programs might not be able to keep up with the demand to produce sufficient numbers of professional nurse graduates. This could created a devastating nursing shortage.

Nurse academics saw the failure to compromise as the fault of reactionary nurses from diploma and associate degree programs. They said these nurses could not tolerate change. In response, the nurse academics were labeled arrogant and naïve regarding the making of public policy. It was believed nurse academics demonstrated a lack of common sense in dealing with the realities of nursing practice and the commanding role of the state in determining licensure policy.

Eventually the NYSNA's 1985 Proposal became a political issue. Nurses in opposition to the 1985 Proposal and the New York Hospital Association, which was also in opposition, sought the support of their political representatives. NYSNA's 1985 Proposal, in the form of the Entry into Practice Bill, was introduced in the N.Y. State Legislature ten consecutive years.(11) The Entry into Practice Bill never became law.

In the mid-1980s, the state of North Dakota actually passed legislation similar to the New York Proposal. The baccalaureate degree became the educational requirement for licensure as a professional nurse; the associate degree became the educational requirement for licensure as a practical nurse. In 2003, this was reversed by new legislation. The new legislation mandated the State Board of Nursing to approve programs of less than four years of study for licensure as a professional nurse and programs of less than two academic years of study for licensure as a practical nurse.(12)

This new legislation sent the North Dakota State Board of Nursing back to square one. Graduates of two-year associate degree programs, three-year diploma programs, along with four-year baccalaureate programs would again be eligible for RN licensure. Educational preparation for licensure as a practical nurse would revert to the traditional twelve-month vocational school preparation.

Why was the ANA unable to maneuver the entry into practice proposal through state legislatures? The primary reason was the negative impact to the fastest growing, largest supplier of graduate nurses eligible for RN licensure—the two-year associate degree program. These programs were an integral part of the community college that sponsored them. The students in these programs were members of the local community. Many graduates of these programs were stable older adults with considerable life experience. Once graduated and licensed as an RN, they stayed and worked in the community in which they were educated and in which they lived.

Men and minorities found these programs attractive. In two academic years they would be eligible for licensure as an RN and a well paying job. Also, in comparison to four-year institutions, the tuition at the community college was easier to negotiate, particularly if you were a single parent. The two-year program had the support of the community. For many communities it was their only source of new nurses eligible for RN licensure. And of course the American Association of Community Colleges (AACN) was a steadfast supporter. From a sociological point of view, the two-year associate degree nursing educational program had a lot going for it. Heaven help the state legislator who would turn these programs into programs for practical nurses. Again, the ANA and the nursing establishment as a whole failed to correctly read the tea leaves.

The ANA 1965 Position Paper on Nursing Education and the 1985 Proposal were attempts to satisfy the dream of professional status for at least some nurses. These futile attempts at influencing the destiny of American nursing were also associated with the sociology of the times. It was a time in America when professional status was synonymous with esteem, financial wellbeing and social status.

It was not only *the* topic of discussion among the nursing academic elite but also among other academics of the day. In 1964, Harold Wilensky of the University of California, Berkeley, noted, "Many occupations engage in heroic struggles for professional identification; few make the grade."(13) More to the point was Fred E. Katz. "Few professionals talk as much about being professionals as those whose professional status is in doubt. Nursing leaders, especially those teaching in university schools of nursing, talk a great deal about being professionals."(14)

American nursing did not benefit from this pursuit for professional standing. Time, energy and focus was averted from more pressing and realistic issues. Solving nursing shortages and devising a rational approach to nursing education and licensing laws were put aside in the quest for professional standing. In 1982, nurse historian Barbara Melosh wrote, "As a strategy for nursing professionalization is doomed to fail; as an ideology, professionalism divides nurses and weds its proponents to limiting and ultimately self-defeating values."(15)

As the century progressed toward the new millenium, the ANA focused less and less on the professional issue. Fewer and fewer references were made to the 1965 Position Paper on Nursing Education. The chief focus of the ANA became their economic security program. The RN designation would continue to be awarded to any graduate of a two-, three- or four-year nursing program who could pass the state administered RN licensure examination. What can be said in conclusion about the 1960s and 1970s and the professional issue? As supplier of the majority of American trained nurses, the associate degree nursing educational program gained significantly in terms of relevance. In contrast, the professional issue lost relevance for most nurses.

References

1. Bixler, Genevieve K. and Ray W. Bixler. "The Professional Status of Nursing." *American Journal of Nursing.* September 1945. pgs. 730–735.

2. Bixler, Genevieve K. and Ray W. Bixler. "The Professional Status of Nursing." *American Journal of Nursing,* August 1959. pgs. 1142–1147.

3. Haase, Patricia T. *The Origins and Rise of Associate Degree Nursing Education.* Durham: Duke University Press. 1990. pg. 121.

4. "Education for Nursing." *American Journal of Nursing.* December 1965. pgs. 106–11.

5. *ibid.* pg. 107–11.

6. Haase. pg. 121.

7. Haase. pg. 122.

8. The 1984 ANA House of Delegates. "Implementation of the Baccalaureate" in *Compendium of Position Statements on Education*. Washington, D.C. American Nurses Publishing. 1995. pg. 41.

9. Kalish, Philip A. and Beatrice J. Kalish. *The Advance of American Nursing*. Philadelphia: J.P. Lippincott Company. 3rd edition. 1995. pgs. 446–7

10. McGriff, Erline and Laura Simms. "Two New York Nurses Debate the NYSNA 1985 Proposal." *American Journal of Nursing*. June 1976. pg. 931.

11. Pavi, Julie M. *Honoring Our Past, Building Our Future.* Franklin, Virginia: Q Publishing. 2000. pg. 156.

12. Mooney, Mary Margaret. "Hog-housed" *Reflections on Nursing Leadership*. Sigma Theta Tau International. 4th Quarter 2003. Volume 29. pg. 8–9.

13. Wilensky, Harold L. "The Professionalization of Everyone." *American Journal of Sociology*. September 1966. pg. 137.

14. Katz. Fred F. "Nurses" in *The Semi-Professions and Their Organization*. Amitai Etzioni, editor. New York: The Free Press. 1969. pg. 71.

15. Melosh, Barbara. *The Physicians Hand: Work Culture and Conflict in American Nursing*. Philadelphia: Temple University Press. 1982. pg. 16.

11

COUNSEL FROM THE PAST

The entry into practice issue was a debacle. Professional status for nurses was a concern only for the nurses in the academic setting. The issue and the concern had created major havoc and divisiveness within nursing. The term "organized nursing" was a misnomer. Any pretense of American nursing functioning as a cohesive occupational force was no longer viable. The perennial unsolved problems of nursing shortages, licensure issues and confusion regarding nursing educational programs remained intact. There was simply no group or organization empowered or even willing to deal with these critical issues.

The nursing establishment was comprised mostly of nurse educators. They had the academic credentials. They published. Their names were in print for all to see and revere. Nurse educators were defined by the professional issue. The maxim that education of professionals takes place in institutions of higher learning was a matter of faith for nurse educators. They became obsessed with the process of nursing education. The pursuit of graduate education for nurses acquired the same fervor as the pursuit of the entry into practice issue. Some nurse educators actually supported a doctoral degree (Ph.D., not M.D.) as the entry level degree for the professional nurse. Another criterion for a profession was an organized body of specialized knowledge. Nursing theorists emerged, identifying frames of reference to explain the what, why, and how of nursing. Another interesting phenomenon took place. Behavioral sciences received increased emphasis in the nursing curriculum. Some suspected the emphasis on behavioral sciences was simply an attempt to gain psychosocial sophistication as a means of courting acceptance in the academic world.(1)

The concept of modern nursing definitely originated with the British. The concept of a college education for the nurse definitely originated with the Americans. There is a bit of irony associated with the American concept. A physician, Richard Olding Beard, initiated the first undergraduate program for nurses in 1909, at the University of Minnesota. Beard respected and admired Hampton-Robb. He agreed with her premise the education of the nurse should be independent of the hospital.

> The university or college should assume the ownership and control of the school, whether it owns or does not own the hospital which serves as the laboratory of the school. It must determine and direct the educational

policy of the school. It must guarantee the fitness of its graduates and the degree or diploma is the best public seal it can set upon their work.(2)

In the early years of the twentieth century, additional collegiate programs were established. Simmons College, Northwestern University, and the Universities of Cincinnati, Michigan, Colorado, Indiana, and Washington established baccalaureate programs.(3) However, they grew slowly in number. Universities were not eager to accept nursing as an academic discipline. One reason was the lack of qualified nurses to teach at the college/university level.(4)

Nurse educators were now playing in the big leagues. Without the graduate degree, specifically the earned doctorate not the M.D. degree, the nurse educator was at a distinct disadvantage. She could not expect the same level of recognition and respect given to other faculty members. This was the situation well into the 1960s, when the federal government made money available specifically for graduate study in nursing. Many nurses took the opportunity offered by the U.S. government, obtained the advanced degrees, and assumed leadership positions in academia and the service sector of the hospital industry. Some nursing leaders became so enamored with the idea of advanced academic preparation for nurses that they advocated a clinical doctorate as the entry into practice requirement. In 1987, Luther Christman, RN, Ph.D., a recognized personality in American Nursing, published an article in the *Nursing Administration Quarterly*.(5) At the time of publication, Christman held the position of vice president for Nursing Affairs and dean of the College of

Nursing at the Rush-Presbyterian-St. Luke's Medical Center at Rush University in Chicago. Christman wrote the article at a time when the nursing establishment and ANA were still recovering from the futile attempt to make the baccalaureate degree the entry into practice requirement. He wrote the following:

> Because of the tremendous rate at which scientific knowledge is accumulating, it is not risky to predict that the clinical doctorate will become the entry level requirement for the practice of nursing. If nurses wish to have parity on the health team, they must have equally rigorous clinical preparation.
>
> Imagine how different the milieu of care will be when every nurse, every patient, every hospital administrator and every physician addresses all nurses as "Doctor."

Christman was not alone in advocating a doctorate for the beginning level of nursing practice. In 1978, Rozella M. Schlotfeldt, RN, Ph.D., published an article in the *Nursing Outlook,* a publication of the National League of Nursing. (6) At time of publication, she was a professor of nursing at Case Western Reserve University. She proposed a doctorate of nursing degree or ND. Schlotfeldt listed a number of reasons that nursing practice required such a degree. The most telling reason was "to reorient the nursing community in ways to hasten the emergence of nursing as a scholarly discipline and a fully autonomous practice profession."

Such were the feelings of grandeur among some nurse academics. However, the majority of nursing educators, both former and contemporary, do not believe the clinical doctorate as the entry level degree for nursing practice is a legitimate or reasonable proposal. The knowledge base required to practice nursing simply does not require a clinical doctorate. From a supply, demand, and monetary point of view the idea was simply preposterous.

Both Christman and Schlotfeldt were discussing the nurse at the entry level, the first position on the nurse totem pole. It was speculated there was a political element that extended beyond the academic scene. Some viewed the degree as a means to greater authority within the healthcare system as a whole.(7) Regardless, the clinical doctorate never took hold as an option for entry into practice. However, the clinical doctorate advocates demonstrated a mindset. Their focus remained tied to the acquisition of professional status via the education route. The advanced degree was the means to that end.

Also, the majority of advocates of advanced degrees for nurses were in influential educational positions. Their focus on graduate education fostered a number of serious problems for nursing in general and specifically for the baccalaureate program. The most compelling problem was the general disdain exhibited by these nurse educators toward the technical/clinical aspects of bedside nursing. In pursuit of academic excellence and academic degrees, nursing faculty drifted away from the clinical situation. They allocated fewer and fewer hours to the clinical area as a learning experience for the student. Consequently, students of nursing at the end of the twentieth century lacked what the students at the beginning of the century had in over-abundance—clinical experience. As always, there was no voice of moderation to tell nursing educators not to throw the baby out with the bath water in the hope of gaining professional status.

Both the Flexner and Bixler criteria for a profession called for a specialized body of knowledge, implying a unique body of knowledge. Nurse academics coveted a unique theoretical base to support their demands for professional standing and to support their presence in the academic setting. To the more pragmatic among the nursing academics, a theory of nursing would provide the basis for curriculum design. The latter is an important variable for examination by agencies that accredit nursing educational programs.

The 1960s and the 1970s saw a proliferation of nursing theories. Taken as an aggregate, nursing theories were definitely eclectic. Faye G. Abdellah identified twenty-one nursing problems as a basis for her theoretical model. Imogene M. King identified goal attainment, "the client" instead of the patient, and the interaction of the personal, interpersonal and social systems as the basis of her theory. Dorothea Orem presented a theory of self-care and subdivided that into a theory of self-care, self-care deficit theory, and the theory of nursing systems. Hildegard Peplau, a psychiatric nurse, developed a theory of interpersonal relations. Perhaps the most esoteric was Martha Rogers and her "unitary man" theory. She offered the following:

> The science of nursing is not a summation of facts and principles drawn from other sources; it is a science of synergistic man—unitary man—characterized by

an organizational conceptual system from which are derived the hypothetical generalizations and unifying principles essential to guide practice.(8)

There are many other nursing theorists, each with their own conceptual basis of nursing practice. The interested reader is referred to *Nursing Theories: Conceptual and Philosophical Foundations*.(9) Characteristically, the nursing establishment failed to reach agreement on a theory of nursing. The issue concerning a nursing theory, or lack of one, consumed a great deal of emotional and intellectual energy on the part of nurse academics. Nursing remains an applied science, continuing to utilize the principles of other academic disciplines to explain the theory and practice of nursing. Nursing should experience no regrets regarding this reality. Many others, such as social work and education, have been doing it for years. There is nothing fraudulent with this arrangement.

The tenacity with which certain issues cling to life in American nursing is rather interesting. The professional issue is a case in point. The nursing establishment, the academic types in particular, are victims of a phenomenon Irving Janis called groupthink.(10) He defined this phenomenon as concurrence-seeking tendencies observed among highly cohesive groups. In the groupthink situation the group is convinced of the righteousness of their cause and/or decision. An idea is presented to the group for agreement, not realistic validation. Unanimity is a critical factor, and this is recognized and adhered to by the membership. God help the group member who fails to recognize this fact.

Groupthink, a defective decision making process, existed in each and every nursing generation throughout the twentieth century. There has always been a core group, usually educators, who espoused the message and passed it, intact, to the succeeding generation. Starting with Hampton-Robb and Nutting, the message was always the same. Move nursing education into the academic setting. Seek your identity as a professional. The validity of the message was never questioned.

In reviewing the written history of American nursing it is striking how little dissension is in evidence regarding this message. It is striking how the nursing establishment was able to maintain this message as a multi-generational issue. Groupthink kept the message consistent. Even in contemporary times the message keeps the nursing establishment from acknowledging a new century has arrived and a new paradigm is needed. The education of nurses must change—radically.

The major failure of the contemporary nursing establishment is the failure to recognize the need for substantial change. Examine the era immediately following WWII to the present time. Montag's two-year program came into existence. She managed change by reducing the educational program from three calendar years to two academic years. The reduction was accomplished mainly by reducing the number of hours allotted to clinical experience. The four-year baccalaureate program managed change by introducing different types of clinical experiences. These new changes supported a curriculum model that focused on prevention, wellness and psychosocial/behavioral concepts. Consequently, this took the student to child and adult daycare settings, wellness clinics, ambulatory care settings, field experiences with social workers, and other innumerable experiences devised by creative clinical instructors. All this was accomplished without lengthening the program but at the expense of caring for the acutely ill hospitalized patient.

There has certainly been substantial growth in graduate educational programs for nurses. In turn, the graduates of these programs assume leadership positions and contribute to maintaining the status quo. While American nursing remained in maintenance mode, there was a universal explosion of knowledge. The post WWII era brought new information to the healthcare scene. The knowledge gained caring for members of the military under wartime conditions was brought to the civilian population and impacted the practice of nursing.

Federal money dedicated to hospital construction, medical research, and medical technology impacted the practice of nursing. New therapies, new surgical procedures, and pharmaceutical advances impacted the practice of nursing. Surgical intensive care units, coronary care units, pediatric intensive care units, and neonatal intensive care units impacted the practice of nursing. The computer impacted the practice of nursing. The best word to describe the nature of this multitudinous impact was *technical*. The nursing establishment did not rise to the occasion. They did not plan for major changes in the nursing educational process. Changes were not demanded by the approving authority for educational programs at the state level, the State Board of Nursing. This did not bode well for the student or the consumer of nursing.

In the last quarter of the twentieth century, the federal government's largess toward the hospital industry came to a halt. Closings and mergers of hospitals became the norm. Nursing staffs were downsized, leaving fewer beds and fewer nurses caring for the sickest of the sick in a very high tech atmosphere. The hospital scene was not the place for a new and inexperienced nurse from any nursing educational program. Also, the image of nursing in general was impacted by negative press accounts of negligent and sometimes criminal behavior. American nursing was losing the public's trust. Why? Part of the problem was a simple matter of the student not finding their nursing identity.

Students of both the two and four-year programs have little opportunity to internalize the intricacies of the hospital scene because of the limited time spent in the clinical area. These neophytes assume a new position with a great deal of anxiety. They have no idea what it means to be a staff nurse. In fact, they have no idea if they really want to be a nurse. They realize they need coaching and considerable on the job training. They realize this intuitively, and it has been reinforced by their teachers. Even though they have passed the state board examination and can write RN following their name, they have considerable learning to accomplish in the practical and technical arena of patient care. Without the mastery of essential skills, they will not reach a level where clinical nursing provides personal satisfaction and identity as a team member. The discomfort becomes so unbearable for some that they leave the hospital scene and seek employment in less stressful situations. They become another failure for nursing education and for American nursing.

American nursing was warned. The 1970 Report
of the National Commission on Nursing and Nursing
Education, *Abstract for Action,* gave warnings and solutions.
The nursing literature even published a few brave souls
who deviated from the groupthink process and discussed
their concerns regarding the education of nurses. In 1972,
an article regarding nursing curriculum appeared in the
Nursing Outlook. Ina Madge Longway, an associate professor
of nursing at Loma Linda University, was the author. She
recorded her concerns for the future.

> Knowledge in nursing and related areas is increasing
> at an accelerating rate and the needs of society are
> changing. Person centered curriculums have already
> shown a great deal of viability and are able, like buffer
> systems, to absorb change. But history teaches that
> eventually the present system will be inadequate. ...
> Perhaps the day of the general practitioner in nursing
> will go the way of the general practitioner in medicine.
> The recommendation of the National Commission for
> the Study of Nursing and Nursing Education—episodic
> and distributive—may well indicate the direction of
> change for the future.(11)

In 1975, Jessie M. Scott, RN, Ph.D., was assistant
surgeon general and director, Division of Nursing, United
States Public Health Service. She said the following:

> We are graduating more nurses now than we did
> ten years ago or fifteen years ago. But we need to
> look at the mix of nursing personnel and skills. When
> we graduated nurses fifteen years ago from hospital

schools, they had immediately marketable skills, they had job specific training. Now we are graduating most of our nurses from nursing programs located in educational institutions. As a result of the move from job-specific training to education regarding concepts and principles of care, they do not have a skill easily marketable immediately. Thus, they are having difficulty shifting into the workforce.(12)

But you know, there are straws in the wind that we really ought to be paying attention to now because the decisions made today won't affect today at all. They'll be felt fifteen, twenty years from now. Maybe that's what we didn't do in 1950, look at the long term implications.(13)

In reference to 1950 in the above paragraph, Scott was referring to Montag's two-year program and implications for the future. Longway and Scott were the exceptions. History demonstrated organized nursing paid little heed to the straws in the wind. Martha Rogers of unitary man fame recorded her feelings about substantial change in the education of nurses. "A massive sweep of stale air, for example, attends the jargon of episodic and distributive put forth in *An Abstract for Action,* the Report of the National Commission for the Study of Nursing and Nursing Education."(14) Rogers made this statement in 1972. At the time she was head of the Division of Nursing Education and professor of education at New York University. She had published several books and was considered a leading nurse theorist. She had influence. Why were Rogers and many others like her so opposed to the

Commission's recommendation regarding the two career pathways?(15) As discussed earlier, it was a matter of power and numbers. A two-track system would eventually produce two types of nurses and two types of nursing practice. The power base of organized nursing would eventually divide, and the division would not necessarily be equal. The reality was the nursing establishment had already created a division with the publication of the Position Paper and the entry into practice issue.

Abstract for Action was published in the 1970s. The concept of episodic and distributive career pathways should be reconsidered. Today the nurse is faced with a very complex work situation and requires an education that meets the demands of a highly advanced technological hospital environment. The present system of nursing education simply does not meet these demands. Nursing in hospitals, long-term care facilities, and even the patient's home are now sites requiring nurses with advanced technical skills. The first consideration must be the safety of the patient, which depends upon a technically competent nurse. The work environment of today's nurse requires a focused, technically astute individual able to recognize and deal with the patient's psychological needs. This is the reality. In 1990 Christine A. Tanner, RN, Ph.D., professor of nursing at Oregon Health Services University, School of Nursing, Portland, wrote of the need for such change.

> Never before in our history have there been such compelling reasons for serious study of our educational programs and for major reform. We continue to struggle with our content-overloaded curricula that

attempt simultaneously to "prepare" nurses
to practice in a biomedically oriented disease-care
system and to educate nurses to be responsible
healthcare professionals committed to the social
changes necessary for health promotion and disease
prevention.(16)

Tanner was saying one program cannot do both.
Tanner was addressing the issue in 1990. Lysaught, in
Abstract for Action, addressed the same issue in the 1970s.
In both instances the nursing establishment remained in
character and failed to respond. Today reasonable people
would agree a major change in the education of nurses
is imperative. Also, the first priority for change is the
education of the nurse for the in-patient setting such
as the hospital or nursing home—the episodic career
pathway.

What specific form should these changes assume? Part
of the answer may be found with a concept first put forth
at the turn of the twentieth century—the central school
idea. In September 1902, Mary E.P. Davis, superintendent
of nurses, Boston Hospital for the Insane, presented a
paper at the annual meeting of the American Society of
Superintendents of Training Schools for Nurses.(17) Davis
was concerned with the quality of education for student
nurses in hospital training programs. She was concerned
the hospitals did not adequately provide the student the
concomitants. "The hospital is the place par excellence to
teach the art of nursing and to practice the science, but
it is not the best place, or even a good place, to teach the
concomitants."(18)

Davis' definition of concomitants was the theoretical courses that form the basis for the practical work. Examples would be anatomy, physiology, chemistry, etc. She proposed the concomitants be taught in a one-year preparatory school, followed by two years at the hospital training school. The preparatory school would be independent of the hospital training school. These preparatory schools or central schools would be established "in or near all the great training school centers."(19)

Today we would probably call this regionalization. Davis viewed the central school as a means of maintaining reasonable costs for both student and the hospital. The central school would hire the best qualified teachers and formulate a curriculum with the assistance of a committee of experts. The central school would be responsible for the didactic portion of the student's learning experience. The hospital training schools would do what they do best; they would train nurses. They would provide and oversee the clinical experience of the student nurse. The preparatory school and the hospital would be separate and distinct. They would issue individual certificates of accomplishment. In September 1903, the *American Journal of Nursing* published an announcement regarding a preparatory course for nurses at Drexel Institute in Philadelphia. (20) In part, the announcement stated the following:

> The conviction among those who have given the matter special attention appears to be that this scientific knowledge could be more advantageously acquired if given independently of the professional

work; … if a preparatory course of training in the scientific branches, a knowledge of which is essential to a fully equipped nurse, should be provided, relief from the pressure upon the women in the first year of the training schools would be obtained, while the standard for the education of nurses would be raised along the whole line.(21)

The above words were recorded over one hundred years ago. These observations remained relevant to hospital diploma programs well into the 1950s. The problems of the early months of the nursing program, the probationary period, were well known and known early in the twentieth century. However, the concept as espoused by Davis and demonstrated by the Drexel Institute was not generally accepted. In the 1950s, student nurses were still taking anatomy, physiology, chemistry and microbiology with some clinical assignments under "pressure cooker" conditions. The nursing history texts have little to say about the central school concept or the Drexel Institute. The idea essentially falls silent in the nursing literature. Why? Again, one looks to Hampton-Robb.

Two years following the Drexel Institute announcement, Isabel Hampton-Robb came forward with a proposal, which was, published in the July 1905 *American Journal of Nursing.* (22) She offered the following:

I would advocate the establishment of central institutes in each state offering a comprehensive theoretical and practical training in general nursing. Such institutes would be independent of any particular hospital, but would be organized and administered through a central committee.

The institute, be it distinctly understood, would have to do not only with preliminary courses in connection with the preparation of candidates, but would be responsible for the entire education in general nursing of accepted candidates.

All diplomas would issue from the nursing institute and not from any one hospital. (23)

In the Hampton-Robb version, the hospital was an affiliating agency; the teaching of students was entirely the domain and responsibility of the central institute. Rather than some control, i.e., the first year, Hampton-Robb demanded complete control of the nursing program. In the Drexel Institute version, the institute had teaching responsibilities for the preparatory portion of the program. The student would move to the jurisdiction of a hospital for the apprenticeship portion of her training.

The central school idea was not realized. The all-or-nothing approach of Hampton-Robb was probably the decisive factor. Another lost opportunity for American nursing. A little flexibility in 1905 could have eased the learning conditions for student nurses of many generations.

Why did Hampton-Robb resist the central school concept as proposed by Mary Davis and the Drexel Institute Program? Davis and the Drexel Institute saw the central school concept, followed by a hospital apprenticeship, as a legitimate means of training student nurses. It was a control issue for Hampton-Robb. To Hampton-Robb, a hospital-sponsored apprenticeship was an anathema. The abuses of the hospital apprenticeship system in relation to the training of student nurses are well documented. Historical documents, nursing texts, and oral histories award validity to the numerous accounts of gross inadequacies. Yes, Hampton-Robb had her reasons. However, her all-or-nothing approach did not serve the student. Hampton-Robb and the fledgling nursing establishment could have controlled an important segment of the student's learning experience if they had acquiesced to the central school idea. As it turned out hospitals maintained control of the entire training program well into the twentieth century. Fast forward to the twenty-first century. The community college becomes the central school for hospital sponsored nurse apprenticeship programs.

The collective psyche of contemporary American nursing is similar to that of an adult who experienced an unhappy childhood. Disturbing memories of an oppressive apprenticeship system are merely suppressed and never completely fade away. Contemporary American nursing stands firmly against such a system and is not inclined to forgive and forget. This stand needs to reexamined. There are safeguards in place today that were non-existent one hundred years ago and even fifty years ago. Government regulations and union work rules exist for the sole purpose of protecting the worker. This is an important consideration when discussing a hospital apprenticeship program for contemporary student nurses.

American nursing is now at a juncture where it needs to consider some facts and proceed to reinvent itself.

It is a new century. It's a new ballgame. Does modern apprenticeship training have a role in nursing education programs patterned toward the episodic career pathway? The answer is a definite yes. From the perspective of the contemporary nursing student, time and money are important variables. Many students are paying for their post-secondary school education well into their working years. They deserve to get their money's worth. For the nursing student this means possessing a reasonable level of clinical skills and self-confidence as a new graduate nurse. The student cannot obtain this with the present system of nursing education.

A central school program, an early twentieth-century proposal, combined with a modern-day apprenticeship program in an acute care in-patient setting is a realistic alternative to the present system. An autonomous central school would provide the theoretical basis for a twenty-first century episodic career pathway first described in *Abstract for Action*. Central school curriculum would be developed in consultation with potential employers from in-patient settings. This was an important step Montag ignored in planning the associate degree program. Upon completion of the central school program, authority and responsibility for the student's learning experience would transfer to the in-patient hospital facility. It is very important the student leave the student role associated with the central school. At this point the nursing student must integrate into the hospital's clinical setting as an apprentice. Integration does not occur in any form in the present system of nursing education. This is the reason why new graduate nurses lack any understanding of what it means to be a staff nurse in the in-patient setting.

The next logical question concerns the readiness of hospital administrators to provide the setting and assume the responsibility of an apprenticeship training program. "What's in it for me?" is a legitimate question. First, the hospital is presently conducting an apprenticeship program of sorts. It is the extended orientation program demanded by all new graduate nurses from any type of nursing educational program. Second, a critical issue for the hospital administrator is staffing. The apprentice nurse would contribute to the staffing of the facility. Such a statement surely causes trepidation among all segments of nursing. However, this is the twenty-first century, and there are effective methods of dealing with worker misuse. Also, the student nurse of the twenty-first century is quite different from the student nurse of Hampton-Robb's era. Like the hospital administrator, the student nurse of today will ask "What's in it for me?" without hesitation and proceed accordingly.

The hospital setting is challenging and can be anxiety-provoking for students in apprentice status or otherwise new to the clinical scene. However, this is the time to learn the high tech skills needed to practice episodic nursing. This is the time to work the evening and night tours of duty, the weekends and holidays. This is the time to learn hospitals are twenty-four/seven operations. This is the time to learn if hospital nursing will be a satisfying career. These types of experiences are not provided under the present nursing educational system. Today's nursing students are fortunate if they experience fifteen clinical hours a week, day duty, Monday through Friday. This latter scenario is not the real world of hospital nursing.

The concept of a central school is a product of the early twentieth century. The idea of two career pathways in nursing, the episodic and distributive, is a product of the 1970s. If adjusted for the twenty-first century, they have considerable merit. Many in organized nursing will label these ideas as reactionary and non-professional in character. As in the past, process issues will arise and if allowed, sabotage any attempt to alter the status quo. Issues concerning licensure will definitely arise. The issue of institutional licensure will resurface. (24) There needs to be an empowered body, probably at the national level, to oversee the process of idea to final implementation.

This chapter concludes with comments regarding the four-year baccalaureate degree nursing program. Following WWII, there was a groundswell of support for the establishment of additional baccalaureate nursing programs on college and university campuses. They brought a measure of prestige to the academic setting. These programs also brought considerable financial assistance from the federal government. Although very expensive to operate, these programs would supposedly solve many prevailing problems. The baccalaureate program would prepare future nursing leaders. The baccalaureate program would better serve American society. These programs would find a solution for the ever-present and always threatening nursing shortage. This belief system extended to hospital board rooms. It was generally believed a baccalaureate-prepared nurse would be better prepared to meet the sociological, psychological, as well as the physiological and physical needs of patients.

As the second half of the twentieth century progressed, these assumptions were accepted as fact by many in nursing, medicine, hospital administration, and American society. However, there is another important fact for consideration. The one available objective measurement of knowledge of basic nursing practice of graduates of all three programs is the National Council Licensure Examination for Registered Nurses (NCLEX-RN)—the RN licensing exam. Statistics compiled by the National Council of State Boards of Nursing do not demonstrate the expected superior performance by graduates of baccalaureate programs.(25)

The baccalaureate nursing education program must define its uniqueness. The ambiguity associated with these programs is striking. There should be no pretense baccalaureate students are being prepared to care for sick individuals in a hospital setting. Only nominal attention is paid to the student's experience in this setting. In fact, the reason the student is provided this very limited experience is to meet a state board eligibility requirement for the RN licensure examination. Baccalaureate programs emphasize health maintenance and disease prevention, which is consistent with the distributive career pathway and does not require an in-patient hospital experience. The program's unique contribution to potential students, the healthcare industry, and American society may be found in the distributive career pathway focus.

Finally, departments or schools of nursing in a college or university setting are among the most expensive of undergraduate programs. Placing faculty in the clinical area with students, even for a limited experience, is very expensive. Narrowing the focus of the baccalaureate program to the distributive career pathway would lessen the financial burden for all concerned.

It must be recognized that the problems of American nursing reside with the way we educate nurses and not the way we treat them. Denial is at play for anyone who insists more money, more staff, more respect, or more weekends off duty will solve the endless dissatisfaction of the American nurse.

It is time to accept the fact the teaching of nurses is essentially different from the teaching of history majors. The college campus is not the appropriate site for the education of students intending to function as nurses in hospitals or other episodic settings. The behavior of contemporary student nurses demonstrates this fact. Many of these students are mature, goal-driven men and women. They quickly recognize a serious void in their educational program; they are provided with limited clinical experience. They lack sufficient opportunity to correlate classroom theory with the clinical situation. Consequently and on their own initiative they seek additional clinical opportunities. Many hospitals fulfill this need by sponsoring a highly structured clinical experience for student nurses. These programs are separate and distinct from the student's clinical experience in their two- or four-year academic program. Of course, there is a price tag for these programs. The hospital provides the student with some financial remuneration and considerable supervision. The eventual payback to the hospital is potential employment of a better prepared beginning graduate nurse. Back to the hospital is the future of American nursing.

References

1. Katz, Fred E. "Nurses" in *The Semi-Professions and their Organization*. Amitai Etaioni, editor. New York: The Free press. 1969. pg. 74–75.

2. Beard, Richard Olding. "The Social, Economic and Educational Status of the Nurse." *American Journal of Nursing*. September 1920. pg. 955.

3. Kalish, Philip A. and Beatrice J. Kalish. *The Advance of American Nursing*. J.B. Lippincott Company. 3rd edition. pg. 246–7.

4. Schwirian, Patricia M. *Professionalization of Nursing*. New York: Lippincott Raven Publishers. 1998. pg. 124.

5. Christman, Luther. "The Future of the Nursing Profession." *Nursing Administration Quarterly*. Winter 1987. pgs. 1–8.

6. Schlotfeldt, Rozella M. "The Professional Doctorate: Rationale and Characteristics." *Nursing Outlook*. May 1978. pgs. 302–311.

7. Grace, Helen K. "The Development of Doctoral Education in Nursing: A Historical Perspective" in *The Nursing Profession*. Norma L. Chaska, editor. New York: McGraw-Hill Company. 1978. pg. 112.

8. Rogers, Martha. "To Be or Not to Be." *Nursing Outlook*. January 1972. pg. 43.

9. *Nursing Theories: Conceptual and Philosophical Foundations.* Suzie Kim Hessock and Ingrid Kollock, editors. New York: Springer Publishing Company. 1999.

10. Janis, Irving L. and Leon Marin. *Decision Making.* New York: The Free Press. 1977. pgs. 129–130.

11. Longway, Ina Madge. "Curriculum Concepts - An Historical Analysis." *Nursing Outlook.* February 1972. pg. 120.

12. "Nurses and Nursing's Issues." *American Journal of Nursing.* October 1975. pg. 1853.

13. *ibid.* pg. 1854.

14. Rogers. "To Be or Not To Be." pg. 45.

15. See Chapter 8 for definitions of episodic and distributive career pathways.

16. Tanner, Christine A. " Reflections on the Curriculum Revolution." *Journal of Nursing Education.* September 1990. pg. 296.

17. Davis, Mary E. "Preparatory Work for Nurses." *American Journal of Nursing.* January 1903. pgs. 256–261.

18. *ibid.* pg. 259.

19. *ibid.*

20. "Preparatory Courses for Nurses Training Schools at Drexel Institute, Philadelphia - First Announcement." *American Journal of Nursing.* September 1903. pgs. 965–968.

21. *ibid.* pg. 965.

22. Hampton-Robb, Isabel. "The Affiliation of Training Schools for Nurses for Educational Purposes." *American Journal of Nursing.* July 1905. pgs. 666–679.

23. *ibid.*

24. Institutional Licensure: A proposal of the 1970s that called for elimination of individual licenses; healthcare personnel would be accommodated under the license

issued to the hospital or other healthcare institutions. Physicians were not included in the proposal.

25. National Council of State Boards of Nursing, Inc. *2002 Licensure and Examination Statistics.* NCSBN Research Brief. Volume 13, November 2003. Published in Chicago, Illinois.

12

WHO SPEAKS FOR THEE?

Who speaks for nurses? "Well, it all depends," says the nurse. "I have many options." These many options are another indication of a serious problem for American nursing. Absent is one organization with sufficient power, prestige and purpose to act as a driving force. Absent is one organization that can put the house in order. Absent is one organization that can speak for American nursing.

In 1893, Hampton-Robb, energetic as usual, went to the Chicago World's Fair. She presented a nursing exhibit at the Hospital and Medical Congress and organized a meeting of directors of schools of nursing. From this meeting evolved the American Society of Superintendents of Training Schools for Nursing, known today as the National League of Nursing (NLN). The purpose of the organization was to set standards for educational programs and membership was extended only to nurse educators.

Eventually Hampton-Robb and colleagues recognized the limitations of such narrow membership eligibility. Instead of expanding the scope and membership of the group, they decided on an additional organization. In 1897 the Nurses Associated Alumnae of the United States and Canada, known today as the American Nurses Association (ANA), became a reality. The purpose of this organization was twofold. The membership would expand to include the worker nurse; the organization would provide resources to obtain legal standing for nurses, i.e., licensure. As the decades progressed the NLN became the point organization for educational matters. The ANA assumed the title of professional organization for nurses. Eventually the ANA would evolve into a labor organization.

Creating two organizations was a mistake and haunts American nursing to this day. Unfortunately, dichotomy in some form is the story of American nursing. It underscores the proclivity of the nursing establishment to separate nursing according to education and practice. In fact, this proclivity went beyond the concept of two organizations. The twentieth century fostered the growth of numerous nursing organizations. The ANA's own website lists nearly ninety.(1) The American Academy of Medical-Surgical Nurses, American Assembly for Men in Nursing, Association of Black Nursing Faculty in Higher Education, National Nursing Staff Development Organization, and Society for Vascular Nursing are just a very few identified in the listing. It seems every system of the human body, from the central nervous system to the reproductive system is represented by some society or association of nurses.

At first glance it appears American nursing developed a sophisticated cadre of organizations. At second glance the chaos within American nursing is evident. The lack of cohesiveness is evident. The internal divisions are evident. The absence of a universal voice is evident. In 1987 the American Academy of Nursing published *The Evolution of Nursing Professional Organizations.*(2) The authors recognized the seriousness of the situation with the following description of the reality.

> The current structure of nursing associations shows highly differentiated and little integrated organizations for representing and controlling the important interests and function of the profession. Increasingly, the profession manifests proliferation of specialty organizations, parallel structures, overlapping functions, and conflicts between nursing leadership and members over goals and approaches. These factors have impeded unified development of the major functions of an organization—the development and setting of standards and the promotion of the interests of its constituents in harmony with its wider environmental context.(3)

The authors were right on target. The state of affairs regarding nursing organizations was marked by confusion, not complexity. Unfortunately, there was no group or organization to turn to and say, "fix it."

The ANA and state boards of nursing were major players in mapping the direction of American nursing during the twentieth century. Regarding the ANA, the first two decades of the twentieth century found the organization embedded with the licensure issue. The ANA survived the Depression intact but emerged as a rather neutral organization, having exerted minimal influence on the work situation of the hospital staff nurse. Following the 1929 Depression, the work life of the hospital staff nurse remained essentially the same. Financial remuneration remained inadequate and working conditions substandard.

> About eighty percent of nurses were still required to live in the hospitals. Three-quarters of nurses had no sick pay, half had no free hospitalization, and two-thirds no pension. Broken schedules, arbitrary dismissals, unpaid overtime, fifty to sixty hour weeks, and unposted schedules continued to exist for most staff nurses.(4)

The ANA professed concerns regarding working conditions of the hospital staff nurse. However, the association was reluctant to engage in any activity considered union-like. The official organ of the ANA, the *American Journal of Nursing*, went on record in 1937 and 1938 against union membership for nurses.(5, 6) The 1938 editorial listed eleven reasons for assuming such a stand. Two of those reasons in particular demonstrated a lack of concern and/or understanding regarding the hospital nurses' situation. The editorials implied the nurse should endure for the sake of the patient. The ANA's stance resembles the pre-Nightingale attitude of the religious who functioned with altruistic motivation.

The ANA stands for the fulfillment of all professional obligations. It cannot therefore recommend or approve membership in any organization which has the power to interfere with a nurse's professional obligation to a patient.

Nursing occupies a unique place in the minds of the people. It is one of respect, even affectionate respect. To our people the nurse is essentially a giver of comfort. This fundamental concept psychologically is at war with the need of the individual nurse for reasonable working conditions and for economic security. It is also at war with the methods of the unions.

WWII heightened the misery of the hospital nurse. Due to military needs, nurses were in short supply on the home front. Hospitals were chronically understaffed. Nurses were still compensated with Depression-era salaries and making less money than women factory workers. Furthermore, when nurses complained about working conditions, they were told they were unpatriotic. The ANA was not responsive to pleas for help from their nurse constituents.(7) Letters to the editor attacked the ANA. Nurses threatened to join the CIO unless the ANA did "less talking and more fighting."(8) Finally, the ANA Economic Security Program was adopted at the 1946 Convention. It has been suggested the ANA acted at this time only because of incipient unionization.(9) Anne Zimmerman, a former president of the ANA, offered the ANA'S version for the late arrival on the collective bargaining scene. Zimmerman blames the constituents.

The manner in which nurses viewed their occupational responsibilities prevented them from tackling the issues of economic and general welfare before 1946.(10)

Fear motivated the ANA response in 1946. The fear concerned significant loss of membership. The leadership of the organization recognized failure to act could possibly be the death knoll for the organization. However, the ANA remained concerned about public and professional image. Insecurity regarding the image issue is confirmed in a 1947 article in the *American Journal of Nursing*.

Utilization of collective bargaining by state nurses associations makes it possible for nurses to be represented in the field of economic security by their professional association, rather than by a non-nurse, non-professional group. ... This means assurance that professional standards will be safeguarded; that we will never lose sight of our important responsibilities in relation to the care of the sick; that we would never be involved in strikes or similar coercive techniques, detrimental to the care of the patient and professional status of the nurse as well; that our leadership will always come from members of our own group; and that we may act, effectively and in full professional dignity, to promote our economic security and the ultimate goal of optimal nursing service to the public.(11)

As noted in the statement there was a no-strike provision. There was also the enactment of the Taft-Hartley Act in 1947 that allowed some hospitals to avoid collective bargaining. Nursing was new at the economic security game and somewhat naive.

> The public—and employers of nurses—have respect for nurses and their professional organizations. They are confident that nurses operating through their own organizations will make no unreasonable demands or employ any measures incompatible with professional status and the care of the sick. This respect and confidence are effective instruments in helping the nurse in her program of economic security.(12)

The ANA's lack of sophistication regarding employer/employee relations and concern for a professional image evolved. The organization's public demeanor changed considerably in five years. In 1952, the ANA was more forceful in advocating their economic security program.

> It is also the obligation of the profession to get over to the public these two basic facts; one, if it wants good medical care and nursing service it will have to pay what is necessary to get it, and two, society must no longer look to nurses to subsidize nursing care in hospitals.(13)

Times were changing. The ANA took appropriate steps for certification as a labor organization under the Labor-Management Relations Act of 1947. The no-strike provision was withdrawn in 1968. The Economic Security Program was renamed the ANA Economic and General Welfare Program. Eventually the organization would deal with the general welfare of the nurse, establish practice standards, formulate a code of ethics, establish an information clearing house and a government affairs department. The association would establish formal relationships with the American Nurses Credentialing Center, the latter certifying nurses in their area of practice. Formal relations would exist with the American Nurses Foundation and the American Academy of Nursing. The former was concerned primarily with nursing research grants, and the latter was best described as a group of identified nurse leaders with advanced academic degrees. The Economic and General Welfare Program was reinvented in the year 2000 and the United American Nurses, AFL-CIO (UAN), became the official labor arm of the ANA. This configuration of relationships is perceived by some as an indication of a great multidimensional organization, meeting the needs of the membership in particular and American society in general. Others could perceive this configuration of relationships as a labor organization burdened with multiple conflicts of interest. For example, a potential conflict of interest could evolve between the national association and the constituent associations that act as collective bargaining agents for some nurses at the state/local level. What would happen if a provision in the code of ethics or a standard of practice became a collective bargaining issue at the local level?

There is another conflict of interest that is not potential but quite real. This conflict originates from the 1965 ANA Position Paper on Nursing Education. The paper identified the baccalaureate degree as the entry level requirement for professional nursing practice. The ANA continues to officially support this position, although in a passive manner. Support cannot be too vigorous for fear of alienating a major segment of the membership—associate degree nurses. In turn, associate degree nurses view the ANA as a bargaining agent and look to the NOADN regarding other career matters. Such internal conflicts are sufficient to prevent the ANA from being or becoming premier in nature or stature. The ANA can represent nurses but not nursing. The ANA cannot assume the much needed universal voice for American nursing.

One wonders about the course of events if the ANA remained steadfast to the founding mothers' goals and operated as a professional organization. The standards issue, particularly for educational programs, might have received the needed clarity that is obviously absent today. Mary Parker Follett (1868–1933) was a contemporary of Hampton-Robb, Nutting and Dock. She was considered an early guru in the field of management and organization. She was quite specific about professional organizations.

A professional association is an association with one object above all others. The members do not come together merely for the pleasure of meeting others of the same occupation; nor do they meet primarily to increase their pecuniary gain, although this may be one of the objects. They have intrinsically joined in order better to perform their function. They meet:

- to establish standards
- to maintain standards
- to improve standards
- to educate the public to appreciate standards

- to protect the public from those individuals who have not attained standards or willfully do not follow them
- to protect individual members of the profession from each other.(14)

American nursing does not have an organization that concerns itself primarily with the issue of standards as enumerated by Follett. Furthermore, American nursing does not have a professional organization as initially envisioned by Hampton-Robb and colleagues.

State boards of nursing had a role, albeit less recognized and discussed than that of the ANA, in the shaping of contemporary American nursing. In order to protect the public, the practice of nursing is regulated by the state, hence state boards of nursing. Each state enacts its own nurse practice act. These acts define the scope of nursing practice, identify who is eligible to practice nursing and under what conditions. The nurse practice act of any given state identifies the requirements for licensure. In general, the state board is concerned with the licensure of the nurse, regulations concerning nursing practice, disciplinary matters and approval of nursing educational programs. The latter function is realized in the following manner.

By demanding particular clinical experience credit or contact hours, and faculty/student ratios, the state boards in effect control the patterns of educational preparation. They may exert an influence regarding attempts to alter or revise curricular.(15)

A survey of state boards of nursing conducted in the mid-1990s found "there is little common agreement on any aspect of basic nursing education."(16) The authors described disparities in mandated curriculum content, mandated faculty/student ratios, mandated hours of clinical experience, the utilization of clinical preceptors, etc. A troubling but not surprising finding is the following:

> In many situations, different requirements exist for various types of programs (BSN, ADN, Diploma). However, these divergent directives all lead to registered nurse licensure. Failure of baccalaureate programs to meet generally more stringent criteria would result in ineligibility for licensure on the part of program graduates. At the same time, graduates of other types of programs (ADN, Diploma) do not need to meet these criteria.(17)

It should be noted the above statement has been the situation since the 1950s. Following the failure of the entry into practice proposal, the nursing establishment has not demonstrated any major concern regarding this reality.

State boards of nursing were reasonably effective in their educational oversight responsibilities until the Montag era, and they then failed to stay the course. In the text *Community College Education for Nursing*, Montag addresses the issue of state boards of nursing. It is obvious she had to shop around to find states that would allow her to proceed with the abbreviated program.

Licensure laws and regulations in the various states
may present obstacles to experimental programs. Since
licensure of graduates must be assured, early discussion
with the appropriate licensing body is imperative.
Application of this criterion to the selection of
cooperating colleges meant that it was necessary
to begin in those states where laws did not prohibit
a nursing program of less than three years. It was
obviously not possible at this time to assure graduates
of anything but licensure within the state in which the
college was located.(18)

New Jersey, Michigan, New York, California, Virginia,
Tennessee, and Utah met Montag's need.(19) The state
boards of nursing in these states apparently failed or
refused to recognize the academic and future occupational
inconsistencies of the associate degree program.

As discussed in an earlier chapter, a few individuals
questioned the academic integrity of Montag's proposal.
However, nursing history texts do not elaborate on this
issue. Thus began the saga of granting the same license
to graduate nurses of different educational programs.
How could this happen? State boards of nursing were
regulatory agencies established to protect the public.
Undoubtedly, a contributing factor could be found in the
composition of state boards of that era. One could ask if
board members had strong educational backgrounds and
a consequent and predominant interest in the *process* of
educating the nurse. Did board members begin to serve
the interests of nurse educators associated with two-year
programs and neglect their oversight responsibilities? Did

a form of regulatory capture and groupthink eventually set the stage for general acceptance of the two-year program by all state boards?

Montag's proposed two-year program was probably an easy sell. After all, Montag was from prestigious Teachers College. However, it is the author's opinion the basic failure of state boards of nursing was and remains the failure to identify a specific nursing educational program as the best preparation to qualify for the state issued RN license.

One can speculate regarding the course of certain events. Suppose one state board of nursing maintained Montag's two-year program was not in the best interests of the student, nursing, or society; the program would better serve the educational needs of the student of practical nursing. Such a stand would have been consistent with reports recommending two levels of nursing education and practice. Unfortunately, this did not happen.

There is a historical relationship between the ANA and state boards of nursing. During WWII a Bureau of State Boards of Nurse Examiners was created to assist states in facilitating the licensing of nurses. In 1945, the bureau was incorporated into the ANA and evolved into the ANA Council of State Boards of Nursing. During the 1970s, the public took issue with perceived conflicts of interest between regulatory boards and professional associations. (20) In 1978, the council withdrew from the ANA and established an autonomous nonprofit body—the National Council of State Boards of Nursing, Inc. (NCSBN).

> The purpose of the NCSBN is to provide an organization through which boards of nursing act and counsel

together on matters of common interest—including the development of licensing examinations in nursing.(21)

Membership is comprised of representatives of individual state boards of nursing. The development of the licensing examination is the council's major contribution to the field of nursing. The council does not have authority over individual state boards. The council is not a potential universal voice for American nursing.

There is a nursing organizational prototype that was once powerful and influential. It was the Nursing Council of National Defense, formed in 1940 in anticipation of WWII. In 1942, the name was changed to the National Nursing Council for War Service. The council was comprised of the major nursing organizations of the era—American Nurses Association, National League of Nursing Education, National Organization for Public Health Nursing, Association of Collegiate Schools of Nursing, and National Association of Colored Graduate Nurses. The council was comprised of nursing service agencies—Nursing Services of the American Red Cross, Federal Children's Bureau, United States Army Nurse Corps, United States Navy Nurse Corps, United States Public Health Services, Nursing Service of the Veterans Administration, and the Nursing Service of the Department of Indian Affairs. The council was a planning agency with the following functions.(22)

1. To determine the role of nurses and nursing in the program of national defense;

2. To unify all nursing activities which are directly or indirectly related to national defense;

3. To study nursing resources; to plan the most effective use of these nursing resources; to provide for necessary increases; and to set up the machinery which insure the quickest possible functioning in case of need;

4. To insure the continuance of the high quality of nursing schools and services in order that effective nursing may be maintained in a national emergency;

5. To act as a clearing house regarding nursing and national defense, and to cooperate with other agencies having related activities and functions.

These functions were characteristic of a high-level organization with a mission. The functions were extremely important to the war effort and to nursing. If the history texts are accurate, the council was quite effective. It was described as having tremendous power derived from a record of success in working with government groups. Following the war, the council eliminated "For War Service" from the title and became known as the National Nursing Council.

The name change caused anxiety within nursing circles.(23) To some, the abbreviated title indicated the council planned to emerge as a powerful oversight body in the post war era. The nursing establishment failed to understand this was just what was needed as the nation approached the second half of the twentieth century.

An organization of this nature would bring integration, cohesiveness, continuity of purpose and a universal voice to American nursing. The council was disbanded in 1948; there was no clamor for its continuance. Another missed opportunity for American nursing.

The functions of the National Nursing Council were formulated in the context of WWII. Consider the functions in the context of the twenty-first century.

1. Determine the role of nurses and nursing in contemporary American society.

2. Unify all activities relating to nursing practice and nursing education.

3. Oversee nursing resources in terms of supply and demand.

4. Oversee and maintain quality of nursing educational programs.

5. Function as a clearinghouse regarding nursing matters and cooperate with agencies having related activities and functions.

These five functions, enumerated in simple declarative sentences, represent the essence of immediate and needed reforms in American nursing. These five functions can be accomplished only by an official and empowered group of individuals willing to sacrifice longstanding assumptions concerning the education and practice of nursing. Their official and empowered status would probably be derived, at least initially, from the federal government.

An empowered National Nursing Council could determine the episodic career pathway as the appropriate educational approach for individuals wishing to prepare for the role as nurses in an in-patient setting. Furthermore, the council could command, structure and implement necessary educational programs to accomplish this objective at the state level. With sufficient authority, an empowered council could command, structure and implement just about any initiative deemed in the best interests of nursing and the society it serves.

The second function, to unify all nursing activities, is an operational function of a centralized authority. The unifying of activities is crucial to the survival of American nursing as representative of the Nightingale prototype. Without a centralized unifying force, American nursing will divide, separate, and become obsolete as the major caregivers of hospitalized patients. A new breed of caregiver will come on the scene. The prototype of this caregiver could be the highly trained corpsman found in the military. The nursing establishment will resist a centralized authority. However, the nursing establishment should realize they never possessed the authority, accountability, or the will to unify and make American nursing a functioning whole.

Function three, overseeing nursing resources in terms of supply and demand, is the first step in understanding the sociological, economic, and educational dynamics associated with the chronic nursing shortage. It is the first step in solving for X. Once the dynamics are understood, the empowered council can initiate appropriate action to alleviate the problem of nursing shortages.

Function four, overseeing and maintaining quality of nursing educational programs, would make the council an accrediting body. Many elite nursing agencies have tried but failed in this important function. State boards of nursing, the National League of Nursing, and the American Association of Colleges of Nursing have participated in the accrediting function. However, they have done so with their own agendas. They all allowed the student's hospital clinical experience to be sacrificed in favor of more academic endeavors. Most importantly, the council can establish standards for nursing educational programs that are consistent with the educational needs of nurses in the twenty-first century.

Finally, the clearinghouse function of the council will evolve into the much needed and potentially powerful universal voice for American nursing. Under this rubric, the council will be identified as the "in" people regarding matters of American nursing. The council will be held highly accountable. The council would answer to the consumer of nursing through an official agency at the federal level. The consumer of nursing, who is a voter, will demand answers to such questions as the cause of chronic nursing shortages and the confusing educational preparation of the nurse. A National Nursing Council would be motivated to find answers to these questions. Such a council requires a uniqueness not available to any other group in American nursing—past or present. This uniqueness would be in the form of basic assumptions and/or core beliefs of council members.

1.   Nursing practice is the essence of nursing and defines educational requirements.

2. The professional status issue is not a relevant issue for consideration by the council.

3. A rational approach can be formulated to meet societies' need for nurses.

4. Implementation of new nursing educational programs, both conventional and innovative, will be based on a rational and demonstrable need.

Accountability for implementation of change has been notoriously lacking throughout the history of twentieth-century American nursing. American nursing is not able to develop and maintain an organization that meets its own increasingly complex needs. American nursing enters a new century in disarray, lacking an organization that can provide a platform to the future. American nursing lacks national leaders. American nursing lacks a future without an empowered National Nursing Council.

References

1. American Nurses Association Website. www.nursingworld.org. 2-27-04.
2. Hegyvary, Sue Thomas et. al. *The Evolution of Nursing Professional* Organizations. Kansas City, Missouri: American Academy of Nursing. 1987.
3. *ibid.* pg. 31.
4. Wagner, David. "The Proletarianization of Nurses in the United States, 1932–1946" in *International Journal of Health Services.* Volume 10, #2. (1980) pg. 277.
5. Editorial. *American Journal of Nursing.* July 1937. pg. 766.
6. Editorial. *American Journal of Nursing.* May 1938. pg. 573.

7. Titus, Shirley. "Economic Facts of Life for Nurses." *American Journal of Nursing.* September 1952. pg. 1110.

8. Wagner. pg. 287.

9. *ibid.* pg. 288.

10. Zimmerman, Ann. "The ANA Economic Security Program in Retrospect." *Nursing Forum.* Volume 10, #3. (1971). pg. 312.

11. "The ANA Economic Security Program." *American Journal of Nursing.* February 1947. pg. 72.

12. *ibid.* pg. 73.

13. Titus. pg. 1111.

14. Fox. Eliot M. and L. Urwick. editors. *Dynamic Administration: The Collected Papers of Mary Parker Follett.* New York: Pittman Publishing Corporation, 2nd edition. 1973. pg. 107

15. Packard, Shiela Polifroni and Helen Shah. "Rules and Regulations Governing Nursing Education." *Journal of Professional Nursing.* Volume 10, #2. (March-April) pg. 92.

16. *ibid.* pg. 103.

17. *ibid.* pg. 102.

18. Montag, Mildred. *Community College Education for Nursing.* New York: McGraw-Hill Book Company, Inc. 1959. pg. 32.

19. *ibid.* pg. 35.

20. "A New Licensing Exam for Nurses." *American Journal of Nursing.* April 1980. pg. 223–26.

21. National Council of State Boards of Nursing Website. www.ncsbn.org. 4-14-04.

22. Roberts, Mary M. *American Nursing.* New York: Macmillian Co. 1954. pg. 304–7.

23. Schutt, Barbara G. "The Recent Past." *American Journal of Nursing.* September 1971. pg. 1785.

13

THE SHORTAGE THING

The issue of chronic nursing shortages and the decline in apprenticeship training for nurses share a common timeframe. "Since the Second World War, we have been so conditioned by the man or woman power needs in nursing that we have developed a conditioned verbal reflex. Just as we couple day with night, right with wrong, and boy with girl, most Americans will react to the word nurse with the label shortage."(1) So stated Jerome Lysaught in 1973.

His words remain accurate in today's context. There has been little respite from the dire predictions of hospital administrators, the nursing establishment, union leaders, and politicians. An unabated looming crisis for American society, because of an existing or pending shortage of nurses, has been the state of affairs for over half a century. The issue and consequent discussion of supply and demand for nurses is constant, decade after decade after decade. It simply will not go away.

1962: A severe shortage of nurses exists in the United States today. It is both quantitative and qualitative. Quantitatively, the shortage makes it impossible to supply hospitals and other health facilities and organizations with sufficient numbers of adequately prepared nurses. Qualitatively, it impairs the effectiveness of nursing care.(2)

1975: For over thirty years there has been persistent complaints of a shortage of professional nurses. Hundreds of articles concerning this problem have been published in hospital, nursing, medical and public-health journals. Even the mass circulation magazines and Sunday newspaper supplements have probed its causes and consequences. Gradually an awareness of the situation has been a part of what John Kenneth Galbraith calls our conventional wisdom.(3)

1983: Over the years, hospitals have grappled with periodic shortages of nurses. But as hospitalized patients have increasingly required more complex nursing care, shortages of nurses have become more difficult to handle. By 1980, high vacancy and turnover rates for registered nurses limited the ability to deliver patient care.(4)

1998: Data from the past decade indicate that the decrease in hospital utilization has yet to result in a decline in aggregate RN employment in hospitals.

To the contrary, ... the number of full-time equivalent RNs employed by community hospitals increased by approximately thirty percent between 1985 and 1994, despite an approximately ten percent decrease in the number of hospital beds.(5)

2001: The health and long-term care systems in the United States rely heavily on the services of nurses, the largest group of healthcare workers. Recent media reports and other accounts have raised concerns about the adequacy of both the current and projected supply of nurses to meet the nation's needs.(6)

2002: How can a healthcare system function effectively without an adequate supply of frontline caregivers? What are the real reasons for the erosions we're seeing in the ranks of our nation's nurses? Is this just another one of nursing's periodic crisis, or does it reflect more serious underlying concerns?(7)

Since the 1950s, American nursing has operated in crisis mode concerning the supply and demand issue. The current literature indicates the crisis continues. Reasons cited are an aging workforce, fewer students entering nursing schools, and dissatisfaction with salary and/or working conditions. A review of the literature back to the 1960s generally enumerates the same explanations. Also, proposed remedies have not changed in the last fifty years.

In 2002, the Robert Wood Johnson Foundation issued a publication about the nursing shortage. The publication discussed issue briefs, national reports and white papers published within the 2000–2001 timeframe. It discussed remedies to alleviate the shortages.(8) Interestingly, the perceived remedies depended on the person offering an opinion. However, there was some universality in responses. Nursing educators recommended infusion of money into nursing education programs, particularly at the graduate level. Nursing administrators cited the need to augment an aging workforce, rectify heavy workloads, a need for more respect and recognition of the nurse, and increased compensation. The hospital staff nurse indicated the need for more respect from employers and physicians, elimination of mandated overtime, no weekend duty, improved nurse-patient staffing ratios, additional support staff, and increased compensation. Union representatives demanded legally mandated nurse-patient staffing ratios.

The pendulum swings and the world turns. With the exception of mandated nurse-patient staffing ratios, a relatively new demand, the remedies cited are perpetual in nature. Why has the nursing establishment, the hospital industry and numerous accrediting and regulatory agencies failed to solve for X? What's going on? The answer stems from the manner in which we collect and utilize statistics, the nature of the quick fixes utilized to deal with this long-standing problem, and the manner in which we educate nurses.

There is a tendency to think, speak, and write in global terms when discussing nursing shortages. A nursing shortage is usually discussed in terms of the nation as a whole. When supply and demand issues are the subjects of a congressional hearing, the numbers go into the millions. ("Supply" generally refers to numbers of nurses employed either full or part time; the term "demand" generally refers to numbers of nurses consumers will employ at various rates of compensation.)(9)

When aggregate needs of the nation are discussed, there is an assumption of homogeneity of need. With few exceptions, such as a nation at war, this is not a correct assumption. Also, a shortage of nurses may only pertain to some regions of the country or specific states. Periodically there is a demonstrated shortage for certain types of nurses such as intensive care nurses, obstetrical nurses, etc. Currently in the United States there is a significant shortage of nursing instructors for undergraduate nursing programs.

There is a tendency to utilize a variety of terms or phrases to describe nursing shortages. One example is to say there is a nursing shortage per 100,000 population. This offers very little information. This can be improved by identifying the number of nurses per 100,000 population per state. This would narrow the field considerably.

The numbers of students entering and graduating from nursing educational programs is a statistic used to predict the future availability of nurses. Nurse vacancy rates, usually cited at the individual hospital level, can be used as an indicator. A progressively higher vacancy rate at a hospital could indicate a chronic nursing shortage in the geographical area. It could also indicate progressively poor personnel policies at that individual hospital. All these indicators are compared with their own historical data for evidence of trends.

There is the issue of staffing norms or number of budgeted nurse positions the facility believes is needed to render optimal nursing care. This is basically a judgment call, and the judgment call is usually for more rather than fewer nurses. When these budgeted positions remain unfilled there develops what one author labels a "sense of shortage." Furthermore, this "sense of shortage" intensifies when the numbers are published for all, including the public, to ponder.(10) Defining a nursing shortage is not an easy task. The General Accounting Office put it unequivocally in the following statement.

> National data are not adequate to describe the nature and extent of nurse workforce shortages, nor are data sufficiently sensitive or current to compare nurse workforce availability across states, specialties or provider types.(11)

Specific advice has recently been rendered to policy makers.

> Different definitions of nursing shortages are not equally reliable in discriminating between hospitals and regions with and without nursing shortages. When faced with reports sounding an alarm about a hospital nursing shortage, policymakers should carefully consider the definition of shortage being used.(12)

The authors also suggest that a common indicator of a nursing shortage "is a message from hospital administrators that they are unable to find nurses to staff their hospitals."(13) Just as all politics is local, some nursing shortages may just be local, requiring a local remedy.

In 1969, Eli Ginzberg, an economist, questioned the ever-present assumption of a nursing shortage.

He questioned how a shortage could exist for over twenty years: "[I]n an open society, an open economy, a 'shortage' cannot continue indefinitely."(14) There is one interesting reality to be acknowledged in this concern about nursing shortages. The ratio of nurses to population has increased throughout the years.

Quick fixes to real or perceived nursing shortages fail to solve but only contribute to the problem. The usual scenario is quite predictable. Local and national newspapers report on the looming crisis in availability of nurses. Pleas are made to the federal government for more money to educate more nurses. Nursing schools recruit, educate and produce more nurses. More graduate nurses arrive on the scene, the shortage abates, and a surplus of nurses eventually emerges. With most nursing positions filled, potential nursing students select a career in another field, thus the start of a new nursing shortage. This has been the pattern since the conclusion of WWII.

Throughout the twentieth century, the federal government has been very generous in support of nursing education. It started in WWI with the establishment of the Army School of Nursing. In 1943, the Bolton Act established the U.S. Cadet Nurse Corps. The Nurse Training Act of 1964 authorized millions of dollars for nursing education, including nursing school construction grants, financial support for all program levels and financial assistance to qualified students. Today it is the Nurse Training Act (Title 8 Public Health Service Act) that continues federal appropriations. The major objective of this financial support is to add to the supply of practicing nurses.

Everyone does not agree with this approach.
In 1994, Lois Friss of the University of Southern California
published an article titled "Nursing Studies Laid End to End
Form a Circle."(15) She made the following observation.

Nearly all studies on the impact of federal funding of
nursing education have reached the same conclusion:
Government programs to subsidize nursing education
do not eliminate hospital nursing vacancies. ...
Contrary to their intended effect, subsidized
educational programs turn out new nurses who
depress the wage rate and drive potential and working
nurses from the market.(16)

Several years earlier Eli Ginzberg made essentially
the same observation. "The worst way to try to improve
economic returns to a group is to continue to increase the
supply."(17) The major fix, infusion of federal money into
educational programs, is not the answer to the shortage.
The reality is nursing shortages have stymied everyone.

The core of the problem is the manner in which we
educate student nurses. We are not educating nurses for
areas of greatest need. Since the conclusion of WWII
we have been educating a generic nurse, one without
elementary expertise in any given area of nursing practice.
This applies to graduates of all programs—associate,
baccalaureate, and remaining diploma programs. American
nursing requires a more focused educational approach,
dictated by the demands of the consumer. Consumer
demands depend on where they receive nursing care.
In most instances it is still the hospital or extended care

setting—the episodic setting. These are the patient care areas primarily impacted by nursing shortages.

These shortages are of great concern because of the immediacy of the patients' needs for nursing care. These are the patient care areas that operate twenty-four/seven. These are the patient care areas that have historical roots with Nightingale in Scutari, the birthplace of modern nursing. The present educational approach does not provide these patient care areas with a stable supply of nurses.

The major focus of nursing education must be the episodic career pattern described in *Abstract for Action* and discussed in earlier chapters. There are two definite advantages to this approach. It would provide a more competent and confident worker, comfortable in the in-patient setting and more likely to remain employed in this setting. Educating for an episodic career pattern, versus a generic career pattern, would provide more valid and reliable statistics. Statistical projections regarding availability of nurses to practice in an in-patient/episodic setting would be more accurate. We would know how many of the new graduates were educated to work in the area of greatest need—the in-patient/episodic setting.

Presently, the estimated number of new graduates entering the workforce each year is of little value because of the lack of focus of educational programs. Many graduates, particularly from the four-year baccalaureate program, seek positions consistent with the distributive career pattern. This reality is a major contributing factor to cyclical nursing shortages. Monitoring and appropriately responding to the number of students entering episodic educational programs would be a positive step in dealing with supply and demand issues, cyclical nursing shortages, and issues of quality in nursing education. This would be an important step in managing the shortage thing. This would be appropriate work for an official oversight body as described in the previous chapter. Establishing control of the educational process and the consequent positive effects was discovered very early in the twentieth century by the medical profession.(18) Placing the focus on educational preparation for episodic nursing practice and dealing effectively with the supply and demand issue would be major accomplishments for American nursing. Attempting such accomplishments would constitute a major challenge to the groupthink mentality of the nursing establishment.

Some reports identify working conditions and working environment as major contributors to chronic nursing shortages. Working conditions are pretty straightforward for acceptance or rejection. Salary, benefit packages, job advancement policies, work schedule, mandated overtime policy, and policy for weekend and holiday duty should be in the employee manual. Woe to any nurse who accepts a nursing position without this information.

Working conditions can be dealt with by a capable personnel department. In some settings there is even assistance and encouragement from labor unions. It is the author's opinion that working conditions are not a major problem or cause shortages of nurses. It is the working environment that contributes to chronic nursing shortages.

The working environment or atmosphere of in-patient settings, particularly hospitals, is not for everyone.

The hospital working environment is tough. Only the physically, psychologically, and technically capable can potentially find this environment a satisfying arena in which to spend one's work life. There are those who meet this criteria and still do not find satisfaction. It probably has something to do with the manner in which a person deals with a complex system. A hospital never shuts down, deals predominantly with life or death issues, has many major actors demanding lead roles in the production, and answers to many oversight bodies. Working in a hospital, for many employees, has immense legal and regulatory implications. The word "accountability" takes on a very special meaning for the hospital practitioner. From the community hospital to the urban, highly affiliated medical center, the story remains essentially the same, differing only in degree. The hospital can be anxiety-provoking for both practitioner and patient.

The nurse is an essential if not *the* essential player in the hospital production. It is not an exaggeration to say everyone but the nursing staff could leave at 5:00 p.m. and patients may not notice. However, if all the nurses left and everyone else stayed, the patients would definitely notice. "The role of the nurse is profoundly affected by her obligation to represent continuity of time and place."(19) Unlike other essential players, e.g., doctors, dieticians, laboratory technicians, building management staff, etc., the nurse must always be available to the patient. The nurse cannot leave the immediate patient environment without proper relief.

The patient care unit of the hospital is the working environment of the nurse. However, the nurse does not control her environment. Many major actors penetrate her domain, each demanding her recognition that their presence and relationship to the patient is legitimate. The nurse acknowledges this legitimacy by doing the bidding of the major actors. This is the way it is, and this is the way it has always been. The following is an excerpt from the *American Journal of Nursing*. It is offered as an example of the nurse's lack of control of the domain in which she is assigned so much responsibility.

In 1922 the New York Academy of Medicine published a preliminary report of its nursing sections survey of New York Hospitals (see AJN 22:603, 1922). This study is significant because it included the first recorded time study of institutional nursing. It uncovered the deeply entrenched but generally unacknowledged hospital practice of permitting far more orders to be written for nursing procedures than could be executed properly by the available nursing staff. This habitual failure of the administrators of nursing services and hospitals to bring this anomaly to the attention of the boards of trustees has undoubtedly been responsible for more poor nursing and lowered nursing morale than any other weakness in American nursing.(20)

The situation today is essentially the same as described so many years ago in the above paragraph, just a little more complex in nature. The description demonstrates the cause of "departure anxiety" that afflicts many nurses at the conclusion of their shift. Nurses frequently describe an internal voice telling them they have failed to do something to or for a patient. That "something" may break through the nurse's awareness at 2:00 a.m., resulting in a phone call to the patient unit. This is an example of what nurses mean when they say the job pervades all aspects of their life. The inner voice is partly responsible for some nurses seeking employment in less anxiety-producing areas of nursing such as distributive nursing practice or nursing education. Some simply abandon the field of nursing. The inner voice is very much a part of the nurse's work environment.

In 2001, the American Medical Association House of Delegates offered Resolution 717 titled "Proposal for Easing the Nursing Shortage." The following is an excerpt from that resolution.

> Whereas, a large amount of skilled nurses' time is currently used in non-patient serving activities writing volumes of notes, reports, surveys and forms, often in duplicate or triplicate for governmental agencies which leave the best and brightest nurses isolated at computers or in staffing rooms filling out reports and unavailable to utilize their skills with patients; therefore be it RESOLVED, that our American Medical Association petition our state and national governments to direct their agencies to review all the paper work in the required reporting that does not jeopardize patient care in order to provide more patient care.(21)

This resolution speaks volumes regarding a serious problem for nurses and the hospital industry as a whole. The resolution speaks to out-of-control documentation requirements. This is a problem having a significant negative impact on a nurse's work environment. The AMA resolution addresses documentation requirements of governmental agencies. There are also documentation requirements of numerous non-governmental oversight bodies. One in particular is the Joint Commission on Accreditation of Health Care Organizations (JCAHO). This is a powerful organization. A hospital needs the JCAHO stamp of approval. Without this approval, the hospital is considered a pariah, stripped of essential governmental funding and prestigious medical education programs. The hospital's very existence may come into question. A major method to determine if a hospital, for this discussion a nursing service, is in compliance with standards enumerated by JCAHO is to examine specific documentation. This specific documentation has guidelines and standards that must be followed to be considered compliant.

The nurse is well aware, because it is emphasized by her supervisor, her patient's chart could be "pulled" for intensive examination by a JCAHO surveyor. Insufficient, incorrect or omitted documentation can have serious consequences for the hospital, the nursing service and the nurse. Therefore, the nurse spends considerable time away from the patient's bedside making the documentation right. Consequently, nurses complain about not having sufficient time with patients and/or being overwhelmed by paperwork. This is a major source of anxiety for the nurse and it brings on that 2:00 a.m. voice saying she forgot to do something important for the patient. The documentation issue contributes significantly to the departure of nurses from the hospital scene. Excessive documentation requirements are an industry-wide problem affecting all hospital practitioners. Such requirements are a major barrier to efficient and safe practice in the hospital setting. It will require resolve on the part of industry leaders to correct this very serious problem.

The unpleasant reality is nursing educational programs are the major impediment to a satisfied and competent nursing workforce. Today's nursing student is not allowed the opportunity to realize the true nature of hospital work. She is not allowed the opportunity to discover, while in student status, if she really wants to be a nurse. An apprentice-type education would provide the student nurse with the opportunity to try a nursing career on for size. If the career fits, the student will adjust and proceed to function in the hospital setting. She will not have to wait for her first position as a graduate nurse to realize if she made the correct career choice.

In 2002, *Boston College Magazine* published an article titled "Who Will Care?"(22) The author quotes a graduate of the Boston College School of Nursing. At time of interview, the BC graduate was a director of quality and care management at a hospital near Boston. She placed causation of the nursing shortage on the rapid closure of hospital diploma programs.

"They eliminated the diploma programs without making any type of adjustment or making provisions for who would provide bedside care."(23) This statement overlooks the fact that the nursing leadership of many generations and notables of many disciplines demanded the closure of hospital diploma programs and movement of the education of nurses into the academic setting. Also quite interesting is the statement regarding who would do the bedside nursing. It seems any adjustments or provisions do not include graduates of the four-year college nursing program. The quotation also supports a point made previously in this narrative. The focus of baccalaureate nursing education is not basic nursing care or episodic nursing practice. Baccalaureate nursing education is generic in nature, with an emphasis toward distributive nursing practice. American society and the hospital industry should not look to baccalaureate nursing education to solve the shortage issue.

References

1. Lysaught, Jerome P. *From Abstract into Action.* New York: McGraw-Hill Book Company. 1973. pg. 4.
2. Report of the Surgeon General's Consultant Group on Nursing. *Toward Quality in Nursing.* Government Printing Office. 1963.
3. Yett, Donald E. *An Economic Analysis of the Nursing Shortage.* Lexington, Massachusetts. D.C. Heath and Company. 1975. pg. 1.
4. National Commission of Nursing. *Summary Report and Recommendations.* Chicago: American Hospital Association. April 1983. pg. 1.
5. Fralic, Maryann F. "How is Demand for Registered Nurses in Hospital Settings Changing"? *Strategies for the Future of Nursing.* Edward O'Neill and Janet Coffman, editors. San Francisco: Jassey-Bass Publishers. 1998. pg. 66.
6. GAO-01-944. *Emerging Nurse Shortages.* July, 2001. pg. 1.

7. Schroeder, Steven A. "A Message from the President of Robert Wood Johnson Foundation" in *The American Nursing Shortage*. Princeton, New Jersey: The Robert Wood Johnson Foundation. 2002. pg. ii.

8. *ibid*. pg. 24.

9. Levine, Eugene. "Nursing Supply and Requirements: The Current Situation and Future Prospects" in *Nursing Personnel and the Changing Health Care System*. Cambridge, Mass: Ballinger Publishers. 1978. pg. 24.

10. Glasser, William. "Nursing Leadership and Policy: Some Cross National Comparisons" *The Nursing Profession: Five Sociological Essays*. Fred Davis, editor. New York: Wiley and Sons. 1965. pg. 33.

11. GAO-01-944. *Emerging Nurse Shortages*. July 2001. pg. 1.

12. Grunbach, Kevin et al. "Measuring Shortages of Hospital Nurses: How do You Know a Hospital with a Nursing Shortage When You See One"? *Medical Care Research and Review*. Volume 58. #4. (December 2000). pg. 388.

13. *ibid*.

14. Ginzberg, Eli. with Mirium Ostow. *Men Money and Medicine* . New York: Columbia University Press. 1969. pg. 163.

15. Friss, Lois. "Nursing Studies Laid End to End form a Circle." *Journal of Health Politics, Policy and Law*. Volume 19. #3. (Fall 1994). pg. 597-631.

16. *ibid*. pg. 618.

17. Ginzberg, Eli. "Facing the Facts and Figures." *American Journal of Nursing*. (December 1987). pg. 1596.

18. Starr, Paul. *The Social Transformation of American Medicine*. New York: Basic Books, Inc. 1982. pg. 112-123.

19. Mauksch, Hans O. "The Organizational Control of Nursing Practice." in *The Nursing Profession: Five Sociological Essays.*

20. Roberts, Mary. *American Nursing.* New York: Macmillan Company. 1954. pg. 177.

21. American Medical Association House of Delegates. Resolution 717. "Proposal for Easing Nursing Shortage." June 16, 2001.

22. Friedman, Gail. "Who Will Care?" *Boston College Magazine.* Volume 62, #2 . (Spring 2002). pg. 30-39.

23. *ibid.* pg. 38.

14

ALWAYS A BRIDESMAID

Resolution of the professional status issue was sought for so long by generations of so many in the nursing establishment. Although they failed to achieve their goal, they fought the good fight. They tried valiantly to conform to the dictums of a profession. They made attempts at a nursing theory. Several were devised but none were chosen.

The demand for original nursing research was another battle cry. Graduate programs in nursing incorporated research design courses into their curriculum. Doctoral programs demanded *original* research as a completion requirement. However, nursing, an applied science, was not involved in original research in the classic sense. The final quest for professional status was made via the nurse practitioner movement and primary nursing. Both concepts were about autonomy for the nurse, a basic characteristic associated with a professional person.

The term "nurse practitioner" (NP) requires explanation. In today's parlance the term is a misnomer. A reasonable person concludes the term refers to one who practices nursing; the one who cares for patients. She is the individual who walks into the hospital room and states, "I am your nurse." This is not the contemporary meaning of the term. The term "nurse practitioner" is employed to identify one's self as separate and distinct from the medical practitioner (MD) and from the individual who practices the traditional Nightingale brand of nursing. The NP is not a nurse in the traditional sense. The NP performs tasks once considered the purview of the physician. She functions in a relatively independent fashion but within guidelines and protocols established by the physician. This is the extent of the coveted autonomy. The NP, like the physician's assistant (PA), is a physician extender. She assists the physician in the office setting, the hospital, or in clinic settings. (The PA programs were started at Duke University in the mid-1960s. Former military corpsmen in particular were attracted to these programs.) Many in nursing vehemently deny the label "physician extender." However, denial does not change reality. The NP is a very valuable member of the healthcare team. Like the PA, she is not an autonomous practitioner.

The first NP program was established at the University of Colorado, also in the mid-1960s. Initially the nursing establishment did not approve of these programs. Martha Rogers of New York University was adamantly opposed. Rogers identified the programs for what they really were—programs to prepare physician extenders. They were "designed to provide succor and profit for the nation's shamans."(1) As discussed earlier, Rogers was dedicated to the belief the nurse was a professional separate and distinct from the physician. She believed nurses who went over to the other side were no longer nurses but assistants to physicians. They were guilty of high treason.

Luther Christman of clinical doctorate for entry level fame viewed the NP program from a positive perspective. He chastised Rogers, the ANA, the NLN and collegiate education regarding their lack of support. "And I believe they did that with more misplaced emotion than reason."(2) The initial negative perspective of the nursing establishment toward NP programs provided the PAs with a head start on their NP colleagues. PA programs flourished, NP programs limped along, and PAs expeditiously found their place in the healthcare industry. They knew who they were and what they wanted to be— an assistant to the physician. In contrast, the NP assumed duties identical to the PA for very different reasons. "The nurse practitioner role offered the promise of greater autonomy, higher status and better economic rewards." (3) The promise of autonomy was not realized. To many in nursing, the NP lost her unique contribution to healthcare by relinquishing her role as direct caregiver and assuming the duties of a mini or lesser doctor.

Primary nursing was the final attempt in the quest for professional status. Successful implementation of primary nursing was surely the answer. Such were the dreams and hopes of many in the world of the nursing establishment, particularly nurse educators in baccalaureate programs. The educators espoused primary nursing as the one true form of nursing suitable for the professional nurse. Student nurses were indoctrinated with this belief system of their instructors. Primary nursing, a hospital-based nursing care delivery system, is characterized by all RN staff holding baccalaureate degrees. Emphasis is placed on the concept of the nurse as an autonomous practitioner. It is in contrast to team nursing, the nursing care delivery system that incorporates ancillary staff such as practical nurses and nursing assistants.

Unlike the NP movement that essentially turned its back on traditional nursing, primary nursing was concerned with issues of control and monopolization of nursing. Practical nurses and nursing assistants would not be players in this nursing care delivery system. These individuals did not meet educational standards. They also represented the continued threat to the RN as the single player in nursing care delivery. Primary nursing was envisioned as the one true professional nursing model. "Primary nursing is a delivery system that creates the opportunity for nurses to develop a truly professional role in hospital nursing today."(4) Nursing administrators, charged with meeting staffing needs for an entire in-patient facility, were divided on the issue of primary nursing. They were very concerned about costs associated with an all RN staff.

The concept of primary nursing was pursued by the nursing establishment on the basis of the professional issue. The concept of primary nursing was sold by the nursing establishment on the assumption that an all RN staff would increase productivity. The RN would no longer be supervising the practical nurse and nursing assistant. The RN would focus entirely on delivery of nursing care, and this would entail the establishment of a therapeutic nurse-patient relationship. In turn the therapeutic nurse-patient relationship would enhance the quality of nursing care. This enhancement would foster a more rapid healing process, effecting an earlier patient discharge from the hospital. A decreased length of stay for the patient was an increase in productivity for the hospital. Some hospital administrators bought into this scenario without objective evidence supporting these claims.

One of the most prestigious medical centers in the country, Beth Israel (BI) in Boston would become the flagship for primary nursing. Primary nursing had a long and acclaimed run at BI. The process started in 1974 and lasted in its purest form to the mid-1990s. Joyce Clifford, RN, Vice President of Nursing, was a major player at BI and the major force and advocate for primary nursing. She and her nursing staff received accolades and personal visits from a worldwide audience of admirers. Clifford was the envy of many of her fellow nursing administrators. She apparently did not have a nurse supply problem even though she hired only nurses with baccalaureate degrees. (It should be noted there are several baccalaureate degree nursing programs in the Boston area.)

And then the unthinkable happened. It was 1995 and BI, an affiliate of Harvard Medical School, experienced serious financial problems. Consequently, BI joined in the merger mania of the decade. It joined with the New England Deaconess, another well known and respected Boston medical center. The merger did not solve the

financial problems of the entity now known as Beth
Israel Deaconess Medical Center (BIDMC), and in 1999
a consultant group was hired to make things right. From
this consultant group came a plan known as Genesis. The
objectives of the plan were to cut costs, increase revenues,
and institute organizational restructuring. Also in 1999,
Clifford assumed the position of chief nurse executive at
CareGroup, the BIDMC parent company. It is implied she
was promoted up and out.(5) Clifford's departure and the
organizational changes at BIDMC impacted the self-image
of the staff nurse. The staff nurse no longer considered
herself a major player in the organization.

BIDMC was losing over a million dollars a week in the
1999 fiscal year. Such extreme loses required dramatic
action. New leadership was in place. It was unclear
whether the values that guided the former Beth Israel,
particularly the pride of place given nursing, would still
be maintained. Nurses' relationships with patients had
become less central as the hospital's leadership's focus
became financial survival and cost-effectiveness.(6)

Primary nursing was unable to meet the financial
strain test and Genesis. Ancillary personnel were added to
the nursing staff, and this in turn decreased the intensity
of the RN's relationship with the patient. The nurse-
patient relationship, a key element in primary nursing, was
impacted by another phenomenon. The patients' average
length of stay decreased significantly. The patient was
discharged as quickly as possible, not providing time for
the establishment of an in-depth nurse-patient relationship.

Primary nursing at BIDMC was essentially dismantled by the fiscal realities of the day. The working environment for the RN changed radically. The attempt to establish the nurse as an autonomous professional person in the hospital setting came to an end.

The concept of autonomy for nurses was the essence of primary nursing in a hospital in-patient setting. Autonomy for the nurse in the hospital setting was essentially a non-starter. Everyone doing their own thing in a complex organization is simply not realistic. Joyce Clifford recognized there were problems with the autonomy issue even at BI. In 1990 she wrote the following:

> While nurses frequently stated they wanted to be autonomous in their practice, or, in other words, they wanted control over their practice, their understanding of these concepts were limited. The notion that their professional autonomy would have boundaries, for example, was foreign to most nurses and the areas in which they often sought freedom of decision making were those that bordered on someone else's area of autonomous practice.(7)

This statement by Clifford, although not intended to be so, was essentially an indictment of baccalaureate nursing education. Educators were fostering the autonomous issue with the naïve student nurse, yet the concept was without application in the real world of nursing. Even Clifford was unable to correlate the concept with the clinical setting. She made an attempt. She identified two types of nurse autonomy—organizational autonomy and clinical practice autonomy. However, she could not make the shoe fit. Consider the following:

> Organizational autonomy represents the opportunity to work in the environment that is free from rules and regulations that have little bearing in the process and outcomes of patient care. Clinical nurses expect to be participants in the decision making process as a whole. They wish to plan their own day, organize their own workload, decide priorities, and in general "control their own practice."(8)

The first part of the definition is ambiguous. There are vague and obscure references to freedom from rules, regulations, and expectations concerning the process of patient care. The latter part of the statement is more definitive and describes an untenable situation in a hospital in-patient setting. Nurses cannot plan their own day in a vacuum. Organizing the workload and setting priorities are dictated by the immediacy of patient demands. Experienced nurses also realize "all hell can break loose" at a moment's notice, and this in turn will dictate demands to the nurse. Essentially the nurse reacts to the demands of the patient care setting.

The following is Clifford's definition of clinical practice autonomy.

> Clinical practice autonomy relates to the scope of practice for which a nurse is accountable. The provision of nursing care to patients is the legitimate area within which nurses believe they have the right to make the decisions. Where the boundaries of nursing practice

overlap with other disciplines, nurses believe they have the right to expect that their knowledge and expertise will be valued in the decision making process.(9)

The first part of the statement is applicable to all nursing practice and consistent with nurse practice acts. The second part of the statement is a request. Clifford is asking members of other disciplines to acknowledge and respect the opinion of the nurse. Such a request is certainly appropriate and is an intrinsic aspect of successful interdisciplinary relationships in any clinical setting. Such relationships are not unique to primary nursing.

Clifford was unable to operationalized the definitions of organizational and clinical practice autonomy. However, the fiscal woes of the 1990s made the issues moot. A great deal has been recorded about primary nursing. Nursing journals abound with articles on the topic. Nursing textbooks deal with the issue in depth and a book for general readership was published in 2003.(10) From all these sources, the key phrase for describing the concept remains "all RN staff." Except for specialty units such as ICUs, the concept of primary nursing is not a viable fiscal option for most hospitals. The concept of primary nursing is more consistent with the practice of nursing in the early twentieth century. Nurses of that era, the private duty and public health nurse, had the greatest degree of autonomy known to practicing nurses. Although there was a physician in the background, these nurses operated with a wide degree of independence. They had time to establish in-depth relationships with their patients. Once nurses entered the hospital as staff nurses the situation changed in an essential manner. Nurses were now employees of an organization, caring for many patients. They were no longer quasi-autonomous practitioners.

Times were changing, not only in Boston but across the entire United States. To deal with the financial crisis, hospital administrators instituted efficiency measures. Accompanying the financial woes of the hospital industry was another cyclical nursing shortage. Many in the nursing establishment blamed this particular shortage on hospital administrators. They believed the fiscal maneuvers in the name of efficiency caused reductions in RN staffing, and this in turn caused major dissatisfaction among nurses, resulting in recruitment problems. Others maintained the cyclical nursing shortage emerged in the late 1980s, before the financial problems of the mid-1990s.

Regardless, fiscal problems combined with a cyclical nursing shortage caused a staffing crisis within the hospital industry. The staffing crisis, as in the past, returned the practical nurse and the nursing assistant to the nursing team. It also brought unrest among hospital nurses. The nurse working in the hospital in-patient setting now sought to command a tailor-made work environment. Issues of professional status, primary nursing, and autonomy gave way to demands for nurse-patient staffing ratios and the elimination of mandated overtime. These demands were supported by labor organizations. The staff nurse was going public with her concerns. Clinical studies claiming mortality rates of hospitalized patients correlated with numbers and level of education of on duty RNs were being published and highlighted by the news media. Old issues gave way to new issues. However, there was one circumstance that did not changed. American nurses entered the twenty-first century in the same manner their predecessors entered the twentieth century—dissatisfied.

Staffing issues, in this context the numbers of nurses scheduled to be on duty at a specific time, remain a perennial problem for nurses in the hospital setting. Because of a number of variables, an exact formula is not available to predict with certainty the number of nurses to schedule for a particular shift. The best the head nurse has at her disposal is experience, general guidelines, the usual activity of the unit, intuition, and flexibility. The experienced head nurse has been there, done that, and is thus able to predict, with a reasonable degree of certainty, the number of nursing staff needed for a specific timeframe on a specific hospital unit. The experienced head nurse knows the level of expertise of her staff, and this is an indicator of numbers of needed staff. The experienced head nurse recognizes certain signs in the physical or emotional behavior of the patients, and this is an indicator of numbers of needed staff. The key word is "experienced."

There are other variables that enter the staffing equation. The type of unit is important. Is this a medical unit, surgical unit, step-down surgical unit, or a neonatal intensive care unit? Is it a medical or surgical intensive care unit (ICU)? Staffing for each of these units varies considerably. Staffing requirements for ICUs are quite specific. Under certain conditions, one nurse to two patients is a common ratio. ICUs are not the most difficult units to staff, providing you have sufficient number of trained ICU nurses. These units are usually smaller in bed capacity.

General medical units are quite challenging from a staffing perspective. In today's financial atmosphere only the very ill may apply. These patients present a variety of physical conditions such as cardiac problems, uncontrolled diabetes, or perhaps the patient requires a blood transfusion or a special procedure. Some patients, although acutely ill, are relatively stable, and much of their care can be accomplished by a practical nurse. Some patients are just a step away from needing an ICU bed, requiring a great deal of the RN's attention. A medically ill psychiatric patient frequently requires a one-to-one situation.

Another variable in staffing consideration is the geographical layout of the unit. What is the configuration of patient rooms in relation to the nurses' station? Do the rooms encircle the nurses' station? Are patient rooms located in corridors jetting out from the nurses' station? Generally speaking, more nursing staff is required for the latter configuration.

Is this a teaching unit? This is a very influential variable. A teaching unit is utilized by doctors in clinical training. These units are usually labeled complex due to level of activity generated by individuals in training. They tend to write more medical orders, consistent with their learning status. These medical orders in turn generate a required action by the nurse. For example, the nurse may have to set up a new medication for the patient, prepare the patient for a test, or prepare the patient for discharge from the hospital. At the very minimum, the nurse would have to engage in some patient teaching.

Fluidity and change are key words in describing ward activity. There is nothing static about a patient care unit.

Patient care units can experience a metamorphosis at a moment's notice. A change in just one patient's condition can dramatically change staffing requirements. A patient may require transfer to the ICU. Multiple staff members will be needed to accompany the patient during transfer. Immediate adjustments must be made to staffing so the remaining patients receive appropriate care. Sometimes other patient care units may be called to send help. This is called "floating" and is very unsettling for all involved. A patient care unit can start the shift with the appropriate complement of staff; one critical patient incident can radically alter staffing requirements.

The staffing issue is emotionally charged and has become cause celebre for organized labor. Why so much emotion? There are a number of reasons. One is the general uncertainty about staffing numbers that prevails in most in-patient/episodic settings. The staffing situation rarely remains stable. This instability can cause that inner voice to reach the nurse's conscious awareness and create havoc with her anxiety level. The voice questions if she can handle the unexpected, which will certainly emerge. She begins to question her own competence. Will I know what to do? Will I make a mistake and harm the patient? Will I do something so egregious I will lose my job and be reported to the State Board of Nursing? These questions cause anxious moments, particularly for the inexperienced nurse.

Then there is the phenomenon known as change. Change is part of the human condition and an intrinsic part of the patient care setting. Currently change in hospitals is in accelerated mode because of today's fiscal environment.

Since the patient's length of stay is shortened considerably, the nurse is constantly getting to know new and sicker patients. Constantly dealing with change and ambiguity is a threatening situation. The associated anxiety focuses on staffing. The rationale is, "I should at least be able to depend on the number of coworkers I can turn to for help."

To some the answer is simply a matter of mandated nurse-patient staffing ratios. Make it a law that there must be so many nurses for so many patients, and the problem will be solved. Such a law became a reality in California in 2002. Ratio laws will not solve the problem. The uniqueness of units and multiple staffing variables defy legislation. Mandated nurse-patient staffing ratios are not practical and very expensive. These two realities will eventually act against the best interests of nursing. Mandated nurse-patient staffing ratios serve no one, least of all the nurse and her patient. The ratio laws are an attempt to bring a level of certainty to a very fluid situation by demanding a tailor-made work environment.

The other issue nurses and organized labor seek to legislate out of existence is mandated overtime. After a busy day at work, most of the time spent on her feet, the nurse is not inclined to remain beyond her scheduled tour of duty. However, the unit's patient census may have increased, a patient's condition may have worsened, or a fellow staff member may have called in sick. The work environment is in a state of flux, and the staffing requirements for the unit are not met. A nurse is told she must remain on duty until a relief person can respond. This is an example of mandated overtime.

The need for mandated overtime is not necessarily caused by a shortage of nurses. The need may be the result of natural and common occurrences in the patient care environment. It happens frequently in twenty-four/seven organizations like hospitals and fire and police departments. It happens in organizations that provide essential services. It goes with the territory. It goes with being a nurse in an in-patient/episodic setting. The hospital, like any other twenty-four/seven organization, cannot function without mandated overtime. The nurse must stay until relieved, and the supervisor must do everything possible to obtain that relief. Walking away from a patient is unethical and can produce serious legal repercussions for the nurse. The majority of nurses would not consider walking away from their patients. However, they do become quite agitated and verbalize their agitation.

There is something called "planned overtime" that may come into play. As the term, suggests overtime is planned in advance as a method of dealing with inadequate staffing. This usually occurs in response to nursing shortages. The problem develops when the person in charge of scheduling knows in advance of a known staffing shortage on a particular tour of duty and fails to schedule needed staff. The plan, sometimes covert, is to cover the shortage by mandating an on-duty nurse to work overtime.

Overtime of this type is unfair and not ethical. It causes a general lack of trust on the part of the nurse toward the employer and produces a negative work environment. Nurses and union representatives have a legitimate complaint when mandated overtime is used in this manner. It is the obligation of hospital administrators and directors of nursing to obtain the needed staff or close the patient care unit. Hospital administrators are reluctant to close units because of financial revenues and potential impact on the community. Attempting to legislate personnel policies relating to staffing ratios and mandated overtime will not bring the desired controlled work environment. The hospital is simply too complex and fluid an organization to respond as intended to laws and regulations of this nature. The best answer to nurse-patient staffing ratios and mandated overtime remains a sufficient number of well trained nursing staff.

Generally speaking, nurse academics do not engage in issues that demand legislation dictating nurse-patient staffing ratios or elimination of mandated overtime. They have essentially remained silent on the issues. Perhaps they believe that because they are academics, they should remain above the fray. However, some have addressed the issue in a peripheral manner in the form of published studies. These studies identify RN staffing and baccalaureate nursing education as major contributing factors to decreased patient mortality and patient safety issues in the hospital situation.

One example is an article published in the September 24, 2003 issue of the *Journal of the American Medical Association* (JAMA) entitled, "Educational Levels of Hospital Nurses and Patient Mortality."(11) The study concluded that hospitals with higher proportion of baccalaureate degree nurses experienced lower mortality rates among surgical patients. The national media quickly took note and published for the general population. The American Association of Colleges of Nursing (AACN) released a response to the study on their website. "AACN Applauds New Study That Confirms Link Between Nursing Education and Patient Mortality Rates" and "Baccalaureate-Prepared Nurses Are Key To Patient Safety, Preventing Deaths."(12)

To the statistically challenged, understanding the presentation of data in this study can be a daunting task. However, even the less than statistically sophisticated may question some aspects of the study's design. Hospitals in the study were located in Pennsylvania. Data was not obtained directly from hospitals utilized in the study; data was obtained from agencies to which the hospitals reported data. Information about patients was obtained from discharge abstracts submitted to the Pennsylvania Health Care Cost Containment Council. Names of nurses were obtained from the Pennsylvania Board of Nursing, and a random sample of these nurses received study surveys. Information from the survey, which included the respondent's educational background and work site, was projected to the respondent's place of employment for comparison with mortality rates at that facility. Of course, only data from nurses who responded to the survey was available for inclusion in the study.

In 2002, the *New England Journal of Medicine* published an article titled " Nurse-Staffing Levels and the Quality of Care in Hospitals."(13) The authors used administrative data from 799 hospitals in 11 different states. The design of the study was complex; the authors dealt with numerous variables. The conclusions supported the positive influence of the RN to the patient's general welfare.

We found consistent evidence of an association between higher levels of staffing by registered nurses and lower rates of adverse outcomes, but no similar evidence related to staffing by licensed practical nurses or aides.(14)

There are problems with studies of this nature. In 1998, an article in *Nursing Research* reviewed multi-institutional studies and concluded, "Overall, these multi-institutional studies provide only weak support for the idea that more professional nurses lead to better patient outcomes."(15)

Contributing to this problem is the reality that nursing does not have standardized databases. This is a serious problem from a research design perspective. There is the real possibility the author of a multi-institutional nursing study is comparing apples with oranges. Multi-institutional studies of the type described are not particularly helpful to nursing or the general public. They tend to contribute to the emotional uproar associated with the looming crisis scenario that is periodically featured in national media. The authors of a *Nursing Research* article put it best.

> Nursing care is a key factor in the outcomes of hospitalized patients, but patient outcomes are also affected by care from other disciplines, the severity and complexity of the patient's condition, other characteristics of the patients, and the work environment. Systematic research addressing these issues has been conducted but suffers from several shortcomings in regard to the relationship of nursing care to patient outcomes.(16)

Nursing cannot be studied in a vacuum. Nurses are not the only workers effecting the patient's wellbeing. Nurses cannot take all the credit for a good patient outcome nor take all the blame when things go terribly wrong for the patient. Good or bad, it is always a team effort.

The story of American nursing is the story of the pursuit of a dream—the professional dream. With all the attempts made to realize that dream, American nursing never arrived at the professional altar. Fortunately the emotion and influence associated with the dream has abated. The resulting void has created an opportunity to produce something real and attainable for the American nurse and the public she serves. This may be the last opportunity to preserve the Nightingale brand of nursing in America. What is needed is an empowered oversight body to implement needed changes. What is needed is a refocusing of nursing education from the generic to the episodic career pathway. What is needed is an American nursing renaissance.

References

1. Rogers, Martha. "Nursing is Coming of Age." *American Journal of Nursing.* (October 1975). pg. 1839.

2. Lysaught, Jerome P. editor. "A Luther Christman Anthology." *Nursing Digest.* Volume 6, #2. (Summer 1978). pg. 14.

3. Aiken, Linda. "Nurses" in *Handbook of Healthcare and the Health Professions.* David Mechanic, editor. New York: The Free Press. 1983. pg. 421.

4. Manthey, Marie. *The Practice of Primary Nursing.* Boston: Blackwell Scientific Publications. 1980. pg. 2.

5. Weinberg, Dana B. *Code Green.* New York: Cornell University Press. 2003. pg. 76.

6. *ibid*. pg. 81.

7. Clifford, Joyce C. "Professionalizing a Nursing Service— An Integrated Approach for the Management of Patient Care" in *Advancing Professional Nursing Practice: Innovations at Boston Beth Israel Hospital*. Joyce Clifford and Kathy Horvath, editors. New York: Springer Publishing Company. 1990. pg. 33.

8. *ibid*. pg. 33.

9. *ibid*. pg. 34.

10. Weinberg.

11. Aiken, Linda H. et al. "Educational Levels of Hospital Nurses and Surgical Patient Mortality." *Journal of American Medical Association*. September 24, 2003. Volume 290. #12. pg. 1617–1633.

12. www.aacn.nche.edu/Media/News Release/2003 AikenStudy.htm.

13. Needleman, Jack. et al. "Nurse Staffing Levels and the Quality of Care in Hospitals." *New England Journal of Medicine*. Volume 346. No. 22. May 30, 2002. pg. 1715–1722.

14. *ibid*. pg. 1720.

15. Biegen, Mary A. et al. "Nurse Staffing and Patient Outcomes." *Nursing Research*. January/February. 1998. pg. 44.

16. *ibid*.

BIBLIOGRAPHY

"A New Licensing Exam for Nurses." *American Journal of Nursing.* April 1980.

Adickes, Sandra L. *To Be Young Was Very Heaven.* New York: St. Martins Press. 1977.

Aiken, Linda. "Nurses" in *Handbook of Healthcare and Health Professions.* David Mechanic, editor. New York: The Free Press. 1983.

Aiken, Linda H. et al. "Educational Levels of Hospital Nurses and Surgical Patient Mortality. *Journal of American Medical Association.* September 24, 2003. Volume 290. #12.

Alcott, Louisa May. *Hospital Sketches.* Reprint of 1863 edition. Chester Connecticut: Applewoods. Distributed by Globe Pequot Press. 1983.

American Medical Association House of Delegates. *Resolution 717. Proposal for Easing Nursing Shortage.* June 16, 2001.

"The ANA Economic Security Program." *American Journal of Nursing.* February 1947.

American Nurses Association Website. www.nursingworld. org. 2-27-04.

Ashley, JoAnn. *Hospitals and the Role of the Nurse.* New York: Teachers College Press. 1979.

Ashley, JoAnn. "Nursing and Early Feminism." *American Journal of Nursing.* September 1975.

Baer, Ellen D. "Nursing's Divided House—an Historical View." *Nursing Research.* Volume 34, # 1. January/February 1985.

Beard, Richard Olding. "The Social, Economic and Educational Status of the Nurse." *American Journal of Nursing.* September 1920.

Biegan, Mary A. et al. "Nurse Staffing and Patient Outcomes." *Nursing Research.* January/February 1998.

Birnbach, Netti and Sandra Lewenson, editors. *First Words: Selected Addresses from the NLN 1894–1933.* New York: National League of Nursing Press. 1991.

Birnbach, Netti and Sandra Lewenson, editors. *Legacy of Leadership: Presidential Addresses from the Superintendents' Society and NLNE, 1894–1952.* New York: National League of Nursing press. 1993.

Bixler, Genevieve K. and Roy W. Bixler. "The Professional Status of Nursing." *American Journal of Nursing.* August 1959.

Bixler, Genevieve K. and Roy W. Bixler. "The Professional Status of Nursing." *American Journal of Nursing.* September 1945.

Brown, Esther Lucille. *Nursing for the Future.* New York: Russell Sage Foundation. 1948.

Buler-Wilkerson, Karen. "False Dawn: the Rise and Decline of Public Health Nursing in America, 1900-1930 in *Nursing History: New Perspectives, New Possibilities.* Ellen c. Lagemann, editor. New York: Teachers College Press. 1983.

Bullough, Bonnie. "The Lasting Impact of World War Two on Nursing." *American Journal of Nursing.* January 1976.

Bullough, Vern L. and Bonnie Bullough. *The Care of the Sick: The Emergence of Modern Nursing.* New York: Prodist. 1978.

Christy, Teresa. "Portrait of a Leader: Isabel Hampton-Robb." *Nursing Outlook.* March 1969.

Christy, Teresa. "Portrait of a Leader: Lavinia Dock." *Nursing Outlook.* June 1969.

Christy, Teresa. "Portrait of a Leader: M. Adelaide Nutting." *Nursing Outlook.* January 1969.

Christy, Teresa., Muriel A Polin and Julie Hover. "An Appraisal of An Abstract for Action." *American Journal of Nursing.* August 1971.

Christian, Luther. "The Future of the Nursing Profession." *Nursing Administration Quarterly.* Winter 1987.

Clappison, Gladys B. *Vassar's Rainbow Division, 1918.* Iowa: The Graphic Publishing Company, Inc. 1964.

Clifford, Joyce C. "Professionalizing a Nursing Service—An Integrated Approach for the Management of Patient Care" in *Advancing Professional Nursing Practice at Boston Beth Israel Hospital.* Joyce Clifford and Kathy Horvarth, editors. New York: Springer Publishing Company. 1990.

Committee on the Function of Nursing. *A Program for the Nursing Profession.* New York: Macmillan Company. 1948.

Committee on the Grading of Nursing Schools. *Nurses, Patients and Pocketbooks. A Report of a Study of the Economics of Nursing.* New York: The Committee. 1928.

Committee for the Study of Nursing Education. *Nursing and Nursing Education in the United States and a Report of a Survey.* Josephine Goldmark, Secretary. New York: The Macmillan Company, 1923.

Davis, Mary F. "Preparatory Work for Nurses." *American Journal of Nursing.* January 1903.

Donahue, Patricia M. *Nursing The Finest Art.* Saint Louis: C.V. Mosby Company. 1985.

Dossey, Barbara Montgomery. *Florence Nightingale: Mystic, Visionary, Healer.* Pennsylvania: Springhouse Corporation. 1999.

Ehrenreich, Barbara L. and Deirdre English. *Witches, Midwives and Nurses: A History of Women Healers.* London: Writers and Readers Publishing Cooperative. 1976.

Editorial. *American Journal of Nursing.* May 1938.

Editorial. *American Journal of Nursing.* July 1937.

Flexner, Abraham. *Is Social Work a Profession?* New York: The New School of Philanthropy. 1915.

Flexner, Abraham. *Medical Education in the United States and Canada. A Report to the Carnegie Fund for the Advancement of Teaching.* New York: Arno Press and the New York Times. 1977.

Fox, Eliot M. and L. Uxoick, editors. *Dynamic Administration: the Collected Papers of Mary Parker Follett.* New York: Pittman Publishing Corporation, 2nd edition. 1973.

Fralic, Maryann F. "How is Demand for Registered Nurses in Hospital Settings Changing"? *Strategies for the Future of Nursing.* Edward O'Neill and Janet Coffman, editors. San Francisco: Jassey-Barr Publishers. 1998.

Friedman, Gail. "Who will Care"? *Boston College Magazine.* Volume 62. #2. Spring 2002.

Fredrickson, George M. *The Inner Civil War.* New York: Harper and Row. 1965.

Friss, Lois. "Nursing Studies Laid End to End Form a Circle." *Journal of Health Politics, Policy and Law.* Volume 19. #3. Fall 1994.

GAO-01-944. *Emerging Nurse Shortages.* July 2001.

Garling, Jean. "Flexner and Goldmark: Why the Difference in Impact?"

Nursing Outlook. Volume 33. #1. January/February 1985.

Garrison, Nancy S. *With Courage and Delicacy.* Mason City, Iowa: Savas Publishing Company. 1999.

Giesberg, Judith Ann. *Civil War Sisterhood.* Boston: Northeastern University Press. 2000.

Ginzberg, Eli. "Facing the Facts and Figures." *American Journal of Nursing.* December 1987.

Ginzberg, Eli. and Mirium Ostow. *Men, Money and Medicine.* New York: Columbia University Press. 1969.

Glasser, William. "Nursing Leadership and Policy: Some Cross National Comparisons." *The Nursing Profession: Five Sociological Essays.* Fred Davis, editor. New York: Wiley & Sons. 1965.

Goldenberg, Gary. *Nurses of a Different Stripe.* New York: Columbia University School of Nursing. 1992.

Goldwater, S.S. "The Nursing Crisis: Efforts to Satisfy the Nursing Requirements of the War. A Way Out of the Difficulty." *American Journal of Nursing.* Volume 18. 1918. Pages 1030–36.

Gould, Louis L., editor. *The Progressive Era.* Syracuse University Press. 1974.

Grace, Helen K. "The Development of Doctoral Education in Nursing. A Historical Perspective" in *The Nursing Profession.* Norma L Chaska, editor. New York: McGraw-Hill Company. 1978.

Grunbach, Kevin et al. "Measuring Shortages of Hospital Nurses: How Do You Know a Hospital with a Nursing Shortage When You See One?" *Medical Care Research and Review.* Volume 58. #4. December 2000.

Haase, Patricia T. *The Origins and Rise of Associate Degree Nursing Education.* Durham: Duke University Press. 1990.

Hampton-Robb, Isabel. "The Affiliation of Training Schools for Nurses for Educational Purposes." *American Journal of Nursing.* July 1905.

Hanson, Kathleen. "The Emergence of Liberal Education in Nursing." *Journal of Professional Nursing.* Volume 5. #2. March/April 1989.

Hegyvary, Sue Thomas. et al. *The Evolution of Nursing Professional Organizations.* Kansas City, Missouri: American Academy of Nursing. 1987.

Irwin, Inez Hayes. *Angels and Amazons.* New York: Doubleday, Doran and Company, Inc. 1933.

James, Janet Wilson, editor. *A Lavinia Dock Reader.* New York: Gailan Publishing Inc. 1985.

James, Janet Wilson. "Isabel Hampton and the Professionalization of Nursing" in *The Therapeutic Revolution.* Morris J. Vogel and Charles F. Rosenberg, editors. Philadelphia: University of Pennsylvania Press. 1979.

Janis, Irving L. and Leon Marin. *Decision Making.* New York: The Free Press. 1977.

Johnson, Dorothy F. *History and Trends of Practical Nursing.* Saint Louis: C.V. Mosby Company. 1966.

Kalish, Philip and Beatrice J. *The Advancement of American Nursing.* Philadelphia: J.B. Lippincott Company. 3rd edition. 1995.

Katz, Fred F. "Nurses" in *The Semi-Professions and Their Organization.* Amitai Etzioni, editor. New York: The Free Press. 1969.

Kernodle, Portia B. *The Red Cross Nurse in Action— 1882–1948.* New York: Harper & Brothers. 1949.

Koch. Harriet B. *Militant Angel.* New York: Macmillan Company. 1951.

Lewenson, Sandra Beth. *Taking Charge: Nursing, Suffrage and Feminism in America 1873–1920*. New York: Garland Publishing. 1983.

Levine, Eugene. "Nursing Supply and Requirements: The Current Situation and Future Prospects" in *Nursing Personnel and the Changing Health Care System*. Cambridge, Mass: Ballinger Publishers. 1978.

Longway, Ina Madge. "Curriculum Concepts—An Historical Analysis." *Nursing Outlook*. February 1972.

Lysaught, Jerome P. editor. "A Luther Christman Anthology." *Nursing Digest*. Volume 6. #2. Summer 1978.

Lysaught, Jerome P. *Abstract in Affirmation*. New York: McGraw-Hill Company. 1981.

Lysaught, Jerome P. *From Abstract into Action*. New York: McGraw-Hill Company. 1973.

Mahaffrey, Elizabeth H. "The Relevance of Associate Degree Nursing Education: Past Present and Future in *On Line Journal of Issues in Nursing*. Volume #7. Manuscript 2. May 31, 2002.

Manthey, Marie. *The Practice of Primary Nursing*. Boston: Blackwell Scientific Publications. 1980.

Marshall, Helen F. *Mary Adelaide Nutting*. Baltimore: John Hopkins University Press. 1972.

Mauksch, Hans O. "The Organizational Control of Nursing Practice" in *The Nursing Profession: Five Sociological Essays*. New York: Wiley and Son. 1965.

May, Ernest R. and the Editors of *Life. The Progressive Era.* Volume 9. 1901–1917. Published by Time Incorporated. 1964.

McClure, Margaret. "Can We Bring Order Out of the Chaos of Nursing Education?" *American Journal of Nursing.* January 1976.

McGriff, Erline and Laura Simms. "Two New York Nurses Debate the NYSNA 1985 Proposal." *American Journal of Nursing.* June 1976.

Melosh, Barbara. *The Physicians Hand.* Philadelphia: Temple University Press. 1982.

Montag, Mildred L. *Community College Education for Nursing.* New York: McGraw-Hill Book Company, Inc. 1959.

Montag, Mildred L. *The Education of Nursing Technicians.* New York: G.P. Putnam & Sons. 1951.

Montag, Mildred L. "Looking Back: Associate Degree Education in Perspective." *Nursing Outlook.* April 1980.

Mooney, Mary Margaret. "Hog-housed" in *Reflections on Nursing Leadership.* Indianapolis: Sigma Theta Tau International. 4th Quarter. 2000. Volume 29.

Moses, Mary. "Why Was NOADN Started?" Closing luncheon speech at meeting of NOADN, Fort Worth. Texas. Novenber 14, 2000.

National Council of State Boards of Nursing, Inc. *2002 Licensure and Examination Statistics.* NCSBN Research Brief. Volume 13. November 2003. Published in Chicago, Illinois.

National League of Nursing. "Report of the Taskforce to Study the Implications of the Recommendations Presented in An Abstract for Action." *Nursing Outlook.* February 1973.

The National Commission for the Study of Nursing and Nursing Education. *Abstract for Action.* Jerome P. Lysaught, Director. New York: McGraw-Hill Company. 1970.

National Commission on Nursing. *Summary Report and Recommendations.* Chicago: American Hospital Association. April 1983.

National Commission of State Boards of Nursing Website. www.ncsbn.org. 4/14/04.

National Research Brief. *2002 Licensure and Examination Statistics.* Chicago, Illinois: National Council of State Boards of Nursing, Inc.

Needlemann, Jack et al. "Nurse Staffing Levels and Quality of Care in Hospitals." *New England Journal of Medicine.* Volume 346. #22. May 30, 2002.

1984 ANA House of Delegates. "Implication of the Baccalaureate" in *Compendium of Position Statements on Education.* Washington, D.C. American Nurses Publishing. 1995.

"Nurses and Nursing Issues." *American Journal of Nursing.* October 1975.

Nursing Theories: Conceptual and Philosophical Foundations. Hesook, Susie Kim and Ingrid Kollock, editors. New York: Springer Publishing Company, 1999.

Nutting, Adelaide M. and Lavinia L Dock. *A History of Nursing.* Volume 2. New York: G.P. Putnam & Sons. 1907.

Nutting, Adelaide M. *A Sound Economic Basis for Schools of Nursing and Other Addresses.* New York: Garland Publishing, Inc. 1984.

O'Brien, Patricia. "All a Woman's Life Can Bring: The Domestic Roots of Nursing in Philadelphia, 1830–1885." *Nursing Research.* January/February, 1987. Volume 36 #1.

Orlick, Annelise. *Common Sense and a Little Fire.* Chapel Hill: University of North Carolina Press. 1995.

Packard, Shiela Polifroni and Helen Shah. "Rules and Regulations Governing Nursing Education. *Journal of Professional Nursing.* Volume 10, #2. March/April.

Parsons, Sara E. *History of the Massachusetts General Hospital Training School for Nurses.* Boston: Whitcomb and Barrows. 1922.

Pavi, Julie M. *Honoring Our Past, Building Our Future.* Franklin, Virginia: Q Publishing. 2000.

Petry, Lucille. "The U.S. Cadet Nurse Corps—A Summing Up." *American Journal of Nursing.* December 1945.

"Preparatory Courses for Nurse Training Schools at Drexel Institute." First Announcement. *American Journal of Nursing.* September 1903.

Report of the Surgeon General's Consultant Group on Nursing. *Toward Quality in Nursing.* Government Printing Office. 1963.

Reverby, Susan. "Something Besides Waiting: the Politics of Private Duty Nursing in the Depression" in *Nursing History: New Perspectives, New Possibilities.* Ellen C. Langeman, editor. New York: Teachers College Press. 1983.

Reverby, Susan. *Ordered to Care.* Cambridge, U.K. Cambridge University Press. 1998.

Richards, Linda. *Reminiscences of Linda Richards.* Boston: Whitcomb and Barrows. 1911.

Roberts, Mary M. *American Nursing.* New York: the Macmillan Company. 1954.

Rogers, Martha. "Nursing Is Coming of Age." *American Journal of Nursing.* October 1975.

Rogers, Martha. "To Be or Not to Be." *Nursing Outlook.* January 1972.

Rosenberg, Charles F. *The Care of Strangers.* New York: Basic Books. 1987.

Safier, Gwendolyn. *Contemporary American Leaders in Nursing.* New York: McGraw Hill Books. 1977.

Schlotfeldt, Rozelle M. "The Professional Doctorate: Rationale and Characteristics. *Nursing Outlook.* May 1978.

Schneider, Dorothy and Carl J. *American Women in the Progressive Era 1900–1920.* New York: Anchor Books, Doubleday. 1993.

Schroeder, Steven A. "A Message from the President of Robert Wood Johnson Foundation" in *American Nursing Shortage.* New Jersey: The Robert Wood Johnson Foundation. 2002.

Schwirian, Patricia M. *Professionalization of Nursing.* New York: Lippincott Raven Publishers. 1998.

Schutt, Barbara G. "The Recent Past." *American Journal of Nursing.* September 1971.

Seymer, Lucy R. *Selected Writings of Florence Nightingale.*
New York: Macmillan Company. 1954.

Shryock, Richard. *The History of Nursing.* Philadelphia:
W.B.Saunders Company. 1959.

Starr, Paul. *The Social Transformation of American Medicine.*
New York: Basic Books, Inc. 1982.

Stimson, Julia C. *Finding Themselves.* New York: the
Macmillan Company. 1918.

Surgeon General's Consultant Group on Nursing. *Toward
Quality in Nursing.* U.S. Department of Health, Education
and Welfare. 1962.

"Surgeon General Looks at Nursing." *American Journal of
Nursing.* January 1967.

Tanner, Christine A. "Reflections on the Curriculum
Revolution." *Journal of Nursing Education.* September 1990.

Titus, Shirley. "Economic Facts of Life for Nurses." *American
Journal of Nursing.* September 1952.

Tomes, Nancy. "The Silent Battle" Nurse Registration
in New York State, 1903–1920" in *Nursing History; New
Perspectives, New Possibilities.* Ellen Lageman, editor. New
York: Teachers College Press. 1983.

Tuckman, Barbara. *Practicing History.* New York: Alfred A.
Knopf. 1981.

United States Public Health Service. *The United States
Cadet Nurse Corps and other Federal Nurse Training Programs.*
Washington, D.C. 1950.

Wagner, David. "The Proletarianization of Nursing in the U.S." *International Journal of Health Services.* Volume 10. #2. 1980.

Weinberg. Dana B. *Code Green.* New York: Cornell University Press. 2003.

Wilensky, Harold L. "The Professionalization of Everyone"? *American Journal of Sociology.* September 1966.

Wolf, Karen. Editor. *JoAnn Ashley: Selected Readings.* New York: National League for Nursing Press. 1977.

www.aacn.nche.edu/Media/NewsRelease/2003/AikenStudy.htm

Yett, Donald E. *An Economic Analysis of the Nursing Shortage.* Lexington, Massachusetts: D.C. Heath and Company. 1975.

Zimmerman, Ann. "The ANA Economic Security Program in Retrospect." *Nursing Forum.* Volume 10. #3. 1971.

INDEX

Abdellah, Faye G. 158
A Program for the Nursing Profession 110–111, 121, 133, 240
Abstract for Action 110, 114, 116–118, 120–122, 163–166, 171, 207, 239, 246
Abstract into Action 119–120, 122, 214, 244
Abstraction in Affirmation 120, 122, 244
academic nurses xiii, 10
Action in nursing 120, 122
Adickes, Sandra 53, 68, 237
Alcott, Louisa May 17, 22, 237
American Academy of Medical-Surgical Nurses 180
American Academy of Nursing 181, 186, 197, 243
American Assembly for Men in Nursing 180
American Association of Colleges of Nursing (AACN) 196, 232

American Association of Community Colleges (AACC) 148
American Federation of Labor (AFL) 92
American Hospital Association (AHA) 66, 78, 98
American Journal of Nursing (AJN) 59, 139, 141, 167, 168, 182, 184, 210
American Medical Association (AMA) 6, 98, 211, 232
American Medical Association House of Delegates 211, 216, 237
American Nursing xii–xv, 1, 3–4, 7–10, 18–20, 23–28, 35–40, 45, 47, 49, 52, 57, 59, 63, 65, 68–69, 71–72, 81, 85, 88, 91–92, 95, 98–102, 106–107, 109–111, 113–116, 118–123, 125–126, 133–136, 141, 143–144, 149, 151, 153, 155, 159–163, 169–170,

175–176, 179–181, 187–188, 192, 194–197, 201, 206, 208, 210, 215–216, 235, 243, 24–8

American Nurses Association (ANA) xiii, 10, 40, 77, 141, 180, 192

American Nurses Association Position Paper on Education for Nursing 141

American Nurses Credentialing Center 186

American Nurses Foundation 186

American Red Cross 72, 74–75, 101–102, 192

American Society of Superintendents of Training Schools for Nurses 39, 166, 179

American Women in the Progressive Era, 1900–1920 52

ANA Council of State Boards of Nursing 191

ANA Economic and General Welfare Program 185

An Appraisal of an Abstract for Action 117, 122, 239

apprentice worker 5

apprenticeship training ix, 41, 103, 171–172, 199

Army Nurse Corps 76–77, 81, 192

Army School of Nursing 75, 77–83, 102, 104, 205

Association of Black Nursing Faculty in Higher Education 180

Autonomy 83, 140, 218–219, 223–226

baccalaureate degree nursing program 173, 221

Barrack Hospital 14

Barton, Clara 17

Beard, Richard Olding 154, 176, 238

Bellevue Hospital 16–17, 24, 26, 75

Bellevue Training School 24–26, 28, 37–38

Beth Israel (BI) 221, 222

Beth Israel Deaconess Medical Center (BIDMC) 222

birth control 29, 52–54

Bixler, Genevieve and Roy 139–140, 150, 158, 238–239

Blackwell, Dr. Elizabeth 16–18, 23–24, 26

Blodgett, Mrs. John 82

Boards of lady Overseers 27

Bolton, Frances Payne 103

Boston City Hospital 30

Boston College xi–xii, 213, 216, 241

Boston Hospital for the Insane 166

Boston Training School 28

Brewster, Mary 56

Brown, Esther Lucille 20, 22, 110, 121, 137, 239

Buehler-Wilkerson, Karen 56, 68, 239

Bureau of State Boards of Nurse Examiners 191

Cadet Nurse Corps 82, 102–104, 108, 205, 247, 249

California State Legislature 45

Carnegie Foundation 47, 93, 107
Case Western Reserve University 156
central school concept 168–169
Chautauqua School of Nursing 64
Christman, Luther 155, 176, 219, 235, 239, 244
Christy, Teresa 36, 48–49, 116, 122, 239
Civil War 4, 17–19, 22–26, 30–31, 36, 40, 72–73, 102, 241
Clifford, Joyce 221, 223, 236, 240
clinical doctorate 155–157, 219
clinical experience x–xi, 5, 64, 127–130, 157, 160, 167, 175, 188–189, 196
Columbia University 9, 38, 45, 73–74, 107, 113, 123, 125, 139, 215, 242
Committee on the Grading of Schools of Nursing 98, 105
Committee of Ladies 24
Community College Education for Nursing 110, 121, 125, 137, 189, 198, 245
Connecticut Training School 28
Congress of Industrial Organizations (CIO) 92
Cooperative Research Project in Junior and Community 125

College Education for Nursing 110, 121, 125, 137, 189, 198, 245
Council of National Defense 78, 192
Council of Nursing Education 82
Crimean War 14, 17, 23, 84

Davis, Mary E.P. 166, 169, 177, 240
Deaconess institute at Kaiserwerth, Germany 13
dean of nursing 75
Delano, Jane 72, 74–78, 85–87
Demock, Susan 30
Department of Veteran Affairs xiv
departure anxiety 210
distributive career pathway/ pattern 117–119, 165, 174–175, 177, 207
Dix, Dorothea Lynde 17
Dock, Lavinia Loyd 31, 33, 36, 38–39, 47–48, 56, 58–61, 68, 87, 92, 239, 243, 246
documentation 10, 110, 117, 211–213
domestic roots of nursing 12, 21, 62, 247
Drexel Institute 167–169, 177, 247
Duke University 137, 150, 218, 242

economic depression of 1873 29
economic security program 150, 183, 185, 198, 238, 250

Educational Levels of Hospital Nurses and Patient Mortality 232

Education of Nursing Technicians 125, 136–137, 245

entry into practice issue 141, 145, 153–154, 165

episodic career pathway/ pattern 116, 166, 171, 195, 207, 235

Evolution of Nursing Professional Organizations 181, 197, 243

Fagin, Claire xiii

Fairleigh Dickinson University 127

Federal Children's Bureau 192

Federal Comstock Laws 53

female garment workers 52, 54, 62

feminists 53, 58

feminist movement 52

Finding Themselves 86, 89, 249

Flexner, Abraham 47, 49, 107, 240, 241

Flexner Report 47, 92–94, 96, 100, 105

Follett, Mary Parker 187, 198, 241

Friss, Lois 206, 215, 241

General Accounting office 204

general media 2–3

Genesis 222

Ginzberg, Eli 110, 112, 119, 133, 146, 204, 206, 215, 241–242

Ginzberg Report 112, 133, 146

Goldenberg, Gary 107, 242

Goldmark Report 94, 96, 110, 112

Goldwater, S.S. 78, 83, 88, 242

Goodrich, Annie 72, 75, 81

Great Depression 9, 57, 91–92, 110

group think 159–160, 163, 191, 208

Harvard Medical School 221

Hassenplug, Lulu K. Wolf 134

healthcare technician 7

Henry Ford Community College 127

Henry Street Settlement 38

Henry Street Visiting Nurse Service 56

Herbert, Sir Henry 14

hospital administrators xiv, 39, 43, 45, 55, 62, 64–65, 83, 92, 130, 172, 199, 204, 221, 226, 231–232

History and Trends of Practical Nursing 85, 89, 108, 243

Hospital and Medical Congress 179

hospital diploma program ix, xi, xiv, 5, 38, 125–126, 130, 144, 146, 168, 213

hospital staff nurse 91–92, 182, 202

Hospital Survey and Construction Act of 1946 (Hill-Burton Act) 124

Howland, Eliza Woolsey 17, 18

Humanitarianism 20

Illinois Training School 37–38

image improvement plan 12, 25
image issue 9, 184
image of nurses 4, 36, 46, 64, 84
influenza epidemic of 1918–19 75
Institute for Nursing Research at Teachers College 125
institutional licensure 173, 177
Is Social Work a Profession 47, 49, 240

Janis, Irving 159, 177, 243
John Hopkins Hospital 37
John Hopkins Training School for Nurses 38
Johnson, Dorothy 85, 89, 108, 243
Joint Commission on Accreditation of Health Care Organizations (JCAHO) 212
Journal of American Medical Association (JAMA) 232

Katz, Fred E. 149, 176
Kernodle, Portia B. 87, 243
King., Imogene M. 158
Koch, Harriet 82, 88, 243

Labor-Management Relations Act of 1947 185
labor movement 7, 9, 45–46, 53, 58, 60, 62, 91–92, 99, 106, 145

lady reformers 23, 26, 36, 123
Lambersten, Eleanor C. 136
legislative initiatives to mandate professional

status 9
Lewenson, Sandra Beth 49, 59, 68, 238, 244
licensure examination 9, 126, 129, 150, 174
licensure of nurses 46, 58
licensed practical nurse (LPN) 101
Lysaught, Jerome 114, 121– 122, 199, 214, 235, 244, 246

mandated overtime 202, 208, 226, 230–232
Massachusetts General Hospital xi, 16, 28, 30, 32, 247
Materia Medica for Nurses 38
McManus, Louise R. 134, 135, 136
Medical Education in the United States and Canada 47, 107, 241
medical establishment 14, 35, 92
Melosh, Barbara 68, 106, 149, 151, 245
Mereness, Dorothy xiii
Mildred's misconception 123–125
Monmouth Memorial Hospital 127
Montag, Mildred 110, 113, 121, 123–127, 129–137, 198, 245
Mother Bickerdyke 17

Mother Evangelist Scholarship Award xi
multi-institutional studies 234

National Association of
   Colored Graduate Nurses
   192
National Commission for the
   Study of Nursing and
   Nursing Education 8, 114,
   121–122, 163–164, 246
National Commission on
   Nursing and Nursing
   Education 110, 163
National Council Licensure
   Examination for Registered
   Nurses (NCLEX-RN) 174
Nursing Council of National
   Defense 192
National Council of State
   Boards of Nursing
   (NCSBN) 109, 174, 178,
   191, 198, 245, 246
National Emergency
   Committee on
   Nursing 73–74
National Joint Practice
   Committee 118
National League of Nursing
   (NLN) 39, 44, 122,
   156, 179, 196, 246
National league of Nursing
   Education (NLNE) 66,
   77, 97, 192
National Nursing Council
   192–197
National Nursing Council for
   War Service 192
national nursing oversight
   council 4

National Nursing Staff
   Development
   organization 180
National Organization for

Public Health Nursing
   77, 192
National Student Defense
   Loans xii
Navy Nurse Corps 74, 192
New England Deaconess 221
New England Hospital for
   Women and Children 16
New England Journal of
   Medicine 233, 236,
   246
New England Training School
   30
New York Hospital 16, 147,
   210
New York State Charities Aid
   Association 24
New York State Nurses
   Association 100, 146
New York University xiii, 164,
   218
Nightingale concept of
   nursing 1
Nightingale, Florence 13, 21,
   83, 240, 249
Nightingale schools 41
Nightingale system 26, 27
   1985 Proposal 145–
   147, 149, 151, 245
1970 Report of National
   Commission on Nursing
   and Nursing Education 163
1963 Vocational Education Act
   144
North Carolina 65, 68, 247
Northwestern University 155

Noyes, Clara D. 66, 87
nurse's aide 72–73, 76, 77, 79,
   85, 86, 100, 102, 105
nurse's aide problem 72, 73

Nurses' Associated Alumnae
of United States and
Canada 39, 40, 180
nurse licensing laws 8
nurse-patient staffing ratios
202, 226, 230, 232
*Nurses Patients and
Pocketbooks* 98, 107,
240
Nurse Practice Act 188, 225
nurse practitioner 217–219
*Nurse Staffing Levels and the
Quality of Care in Hospitals*
233, 236, 246
Nurse Training Act of 1943
(Bolton Act) 103
Nurse Training Act of 1964
205
Nursing Administration Quarterly
155, 176, 239
*Nursing and Nursing Education in
the United States* 94,
107, 240
Nursing for the Future 20–22,
110, 121, 126, 133,
137, 239
nursing curriculum 5–6, 12, 109,
154, 163
nursing establishment xiii, 4, 7, 9,
12, 21, 27–28, 35–36,
40, 42–43, 45–48,
55–59, 61–63, 65,
67, 73, 77, 80, 82, 84–
86, 91, 93–96, 99–100,
102, 105–106, 109,
111–114, 116–121,
126, 131, 140, 145,
149, 153, 156, 159–
161, 165–166, 170,
180, 189, 193, 195,
199, 202, 208, 217–

220, 226
Nursing Outlook 48, 107, 137,
156, 163, 176–177, 239,
241, 244–246, 248
Nursing Research 22, 33, 125,
140, 186, 217, 234, 236, 238,
247
Nursing Service of the
American Red Cross 192
Nursing Service of
Department of Indian
Affairs 192
Nursing Service of the
Veterans
Administration 192
nursing shortage xii, xiv, 1–3,
6, 9–10, 101–102, 113–114,
124, 147, 149, 153, 173,
195–196, 199, 201–208,
211, 213–216, 226, 231,
237, 242, 248, 250
*Nursing Studies Laid End to End
Form a Circle* 206,
215, 241
nursing technician 124, 125,
127, 136–137, 145
Nutting, M. Adelaide 31, 36,
38–39, 42, 45, 47, 49, 72–73,
76–77, 80, 82–83, 94,
98–101, 103, 105, 109, 133,
187, 239

Office of Civilian Defense 102
Orange County Community
College 127
Orem, Dorothea 158
organized labor 7, 229–230

Parsons, Sara E. 28, 32, 247
Pasadena City College 127
patient care provider 7

Pennsylvania Board of Nursing 233
Pennsylvania Health Care Cost Containment Council 233
Pennsylvania Hospital 16, 75
Peplau, Hildegard 158
Pepper, Jessie Mae xiii
persona of victim 63
physician's assistant 20, 218
physician extender 218–219
planned overtime 231
primary nursing 9, 44, 217, 219–223, 225–226, 235, 244
private duty nurses xii, 4, 65
professional issue vii, xii–xiii, xv, 60, 99, 139, 150, 159, 220
professional nurses xi–xii, 60, 80, 86, 111, 142–143, 146, 200, 234
professional status xiii, 7, 9, 36, 37, 39, 42, 47–48, 55, 63, 67, 83, 106, 139–141, 149–150, 153, 157–158, 184–185, 197, 217, 219, 226, 238–239
professional status issue 36, 42, 47, 141, 197, 217
Progressive Era 8, 51–54, 57, 60–61, 63, 67, 72, 99, 242, 245, 248
Providence College x
pseudo professionalism 62
puerperal fever 25

registered care technologist 6
regulatory capture 191
religious orders 12, 17, 29
Richards, Linda 30–32, 87, 248

Reminiscences of Linda Richards 30, 32, 248
Reverby, Susan 68–69, 107, 247–248
Robb, Isabel Hampton 36–43, 45–49, 72, 133, 168–170, 177, 179–180, 187, 239, 242
Robert Wood Johnson Foundation 8, 201, 215, 248
Roberts, Mary 49, 81, 88, 107, 122, 198, 216, 248
Rockefeller Foundation 8, 94
Rogers, Martha xiii, 158, 164, 176, 218, 235, 248
Rosenberg, Charles 22, 26, 32, 49, 248
Rush University 156
Russell, James Earl 45
Russell Sage Foundation 8, 22, 110, 121, 137, 239
Russell, William Howard 14

Sairey Gamps 15
Sanger, Margaret 54
Schlotfeldt, Rozella M. 156, 176, 248
Schneider, Dorothy and Carl 52, 67, 248
Schuyler, Louise 17, 24
Scott, Jessie M. 163
Scutari 14, 207
secular nursing 15, 17, 19, 21
Shryock, Richard 19, 22, 29, 32, 249
Simmons College 155
Sisters of Charity 14
Smith, Dr. Winford 78
societal perception of nurse 4

Society for Vascular Nursing 180

Spanish American War 26

staff nurse xi, 2, 5, 7, 44, 91–92, 99, 103, 162, 172, 182, 202, 222, 225–226

staffing guidelines 3

state board examination xi, 162

St. Joseph's Hospital v, ix

St. Thomas Hospital in London 15, 27

state boards of nursing 2, 7, 10, 44–45, 65, 109, 126, 135–136, 174, 178, 181, 188–192, 196, 198, 245, 246

state legislatures 59, 141, 148

state licensing laws 142, 144

Stimson, Julia C. 86, 89, 249

Stipends 42–43

suffrage 7, 39, 52, 58–60, 68, 244

suffragettes 52–53

Surgeon General's Consultant Group on Nursing 110, 113, 121–122, 214, 247, 249

Surgeon General Gorgas 79

Surgeon General of United States 104, 133

survey course in nursing 6

Taft-Hartley Act 184

Taking Charge: Nursing, Suffrage and Feminism 59, 68, 244

Tanner, Christine A. 165, 177, 249

Tarbell, Ida 51

Teachers College, Columbia University 9, 38, 45, 73, 113, 123, 125

team nursing 220

technical nurse 125, 127, 130–133, 145

ten-day women 16

The Care of Strangers 22, 26, 32, 49, 248

The Militant Angel 82

theory of interpersonal relations 158

theory of nursing 140, 158–159

Thompson, Dora 76

To Be Young Was Very Heaven 53, 68, 237

Tomes, Nancy 69, 249

transport women 18

Triangle Shirtwaist Fire 54

Toward Quality Nursing 110

twenty-four/seven operations 172

two-year associate degree nursing programs xiv, 1, 9, 113, 123, 129, 144

unitary man theory 158

United American Nurses AFL-CIO 186

United States Public Health Services 192

United States Sanitary Commission (USSC) 18

University of California, Berkley 149

University of Cincinnati 155

University of Colorado 218

University of Indiana 155

University of Michigan 155

University of Minnesota 72, 154

University of Pennsylvania
    Hospital School of Nursing
    75
University of Rochester 114
University of Washington 155

Virginia Intermont College
    127
Virginia State College 127
Voluntary Aid Detachments
    85
Vassar College 82
Vassar Training Camp for
    Nurses 82

Wald, Lillian D. 56
Walter Reed General
    Hospital 81
War Nursing Council 101
Warrington, Joseph and Nurse
    Society of
    Philadelphia 16
Weber College 127
White Plains Hospital 54
Wilensky, Harold R. 149
W.K. Kellogg Foundation 120
women reformers 20, 23
Women's Educational
    Association 28
Women's Hospital 37
Women's Rights Convention
    in Seneca Falls 52
Woolsey, Georgeanna 17, 28
working conditions 3, 7, 9, 54,
    67, 92, 99, 182–183,
    201, 208
working environment 208–
    209, 223
World War 1 51, 83–84
World War 2 108

Yale University School of
    Nursing 75

Zakrzewska, Dr. Marie 16
Zimmerman, Anna 183, 198,
    250

Made in the USA
Lexington, KY
12 December 2009